ANTI-INFLAMMATORY DIET MEAL PREP

Heal the Immune System With a Healthy Diet to Stay fit and Feeling Good, Longevity Diet for Everyone.

Emil C. Johnson

Table of Contents

Chapter 10: Creating Your Own Meal Plan............147

Chapter 11: Bonus Tips and Tricks to Sticking to Your Diet 159

Introduction

Your body is meant to function as a sort of automatic machine. It is meant to do everything that you will need for you so that you will be able to live. It has its own built-in regulatory systems. It works with its own personal defense system as well, which is meant to keep you safe and free from harm. Your immune system functions to ensure that at the end of the day, you have everything that you are going to need to function. It ensures that you are in a position where you can and will be able to fend off injuries or illnesses, taking out foreign invaders.

However, sometimes, this immune system doesn't function as intended. Sometimes, it attacks your body instead of defending it, and the end result is inflammation. Inflammation can spread throughout the whole body and cause a whole wide range of issues, from causing problems with your digestive system to your brain, heart, or other organs. As inflammation builds up in your body, it often worsens and causes all sorts of issues for your body as well. You could have symptoms of inflammation in the digestive system that manifest as irritable bowel syndrome. You could find yourself reacting to the inflammation that then causes you to develop diabetes. You could find yourself struggling with other issues as well, and it all comes down to inflammation in the body.

If you are already prone to inflammation issues, then your diet is more important than ever. The foods that you eat will help you to alter how your body functions. After all, the foods that you consume will directly influence how your body functions. When you eat foods that are naturally inflammatory for you, you will struggle. Likewise, when you eat foods that are naturally anti-inflammatory, you will see that your body usually responds by alleviating that inflammation that was occurring throughout the body. For this reason, many people swear by anti-inflammatory diets such as the Mediterranean diet to help themselves control and influence the body to allow for inflammation to be healed.

As you read through this book, you will find yourself discovering all sorts of information about how you can begin to follow the various anti-inflammatory diets for yourself. You will start to see how you can begin to clean up the foods that you consume so that you will be able to be effective in treating your symptoms. When you learn to eat the foods that will help you, your body will be so much better.

When it comes down to it, you are able to influence your body by managing yourself with food. When you eat the right foods, you discover that ultimately, your body is within your control, and it won't take you much at all to manage it. All you have to do is know what you are doing and why. You have to pay attention to the foods you consume, and when you start balancing them out, you will realize that ultimately you can feel better. You can take control of your life and make the changes that will help you. Food is fuel, and the kind of fuel that you feed yourself matters. All you will have to do is figure out how to provide yourself the right fuel to stay healthy and strong.

Keep in mind that this diet is not designed to provide you with a way to lose weight. Though you can lose weight on the anti-inflammatory diet, that is not the primary purpose of following it. Rather, the most compelling reasons for following this diet are all surrounding the idea of inflammation and alleviating it. All that matters for you are figuring out how you can and will be able to cut down on those foods that are going to cause you problems.

Now, you might think that this is going to be highly difficult to follow or that you are going to run into issues with maintaining your diet as you eat these foods. However, that's not true at all, especially if you start implementing meal planning. As you begin to plan your meals accordingly, you will start realizing that you can even enjoy the foods that you consume, and that will allow you to begin eating better than ever with ease. We will also be diving right into the idea of meal planning, working hard to identify what it is that you will need to do to ensure that you stick to your meals accordingly and to ensure that you have all of the groceries on hand at any point in time.

Chapter 1:
Food and Inflammation – Are They Really Related?

As we begin, the most important starting point is figuring out the relationship between food and inflammation. While many people might be quick to tell you that no, they are not connected at all, the truth is that everything in your body relates back to your body in one way or another. It is essential for you to recognize this so that you will be able to provide for yourself. If you want to be able to treat your own body, then you want to ensure that you are managing your inflammation the right way, and food is one of the easiest to manage.

As you read through this chapter, we have a few important topics to consider. We will first go over what inflammation is and how it works in the body. We will also address what causes inflammation and explore the relationship between inflammation and the diet that you consume. We will take the time to address the consequences of inflammation in the body, and finally, address the signs that your body may be actively currently suffering from it.

If you are like many other millions of people, you may find that inflammation is a part of your life that is a bane to your existence. It is uncomfortable. It is unpleasant and painful, and it can manifest in ways that are going to be problematic for you, and because of that, you probably want to find ways that you can better regulate it. That is what you are here for, and the more that you read, the more that you will find the ways to do so!

What Is Inflammation?

To begin understanding how this diet works and what it will do for you, you have to first begin looking at how inflammation impacts the body. Inflammation itself is the process through which your body will produce white blood cells so that the blood cells will be able to protect your body from foreign invaders. The inflammatory process occurs to protect your body from bacteria and viruses that might get into the body through wounds or when you are eating. It also works to protect your body from damage caused as well. By protecting the body from inflammation, you can begin to heal.

However, inflammation isn't all good. Some diseases cause your body's immune system to create inflammation despite there being nothing to ward off in the first place. This is known as an autoimmune disease, and it occurs when the body decides to attack itself rather than any issues. Your body will treat regular tissue as if it is a problem or as if they are infected with something. Typically, inflammation is triggered either chronically or acutely. Acute inflammation is considered short-lived inflammation that will not be there for very long at all. Chronic inflammation will last significantly longer. It will create conditions such as cancer or heart disease. Acute inflammation is short-lived and will not last much longer than a few days, or even weeks at times. However, it is going to fade away at some point.

Inflammation is typically characterized by very easily noticeable symptoms, such as:

- Redness

- Swelling

- Pain in the inflamed area

- Joint stiffness

- Fever

- Fatigue

- Chills

- Headaches

- Lacking appetite

What Causes Inflammation?

Typically, inflammation happens due to chemicals in your white blood cells entering blood or other tissues to protect them from invaders. As a result, the blood flow is raised in that particular area, which causes the increased warmth and redness that is characteristic. Additionally, as the chemicals cause fluids to fill the tissues, swelling is triggered. As swelling happens, many of the nerves may cause pain when they are triggered. The higher the numbers of cells, the more likely you are to have a serious level of inflammation.

Typically, acute inflammation is caused by several different triggers. It could be the case that you suffer from inflammation from causes such as:

- Being exposed to something that is irritating, such as being stung by a bee or inhaling dust or getting something in the eye.

- Being injured and having the local area around the injury swell as the body tries to treat it.

- Infection is present in the area in the body that is beginning to grow inflamed.

When the body starts to trigger an allergic reaction, it then creates the commonly known signs of inflammation. It is likely that the tissues will swell up as proteins are accumulated in the tissue. These acute symptoms are usually not a big deal—inflammation is meant to be acute, and it shows that the body is working.

Chronic inflammation, on the other hand, is much more problematic. Because chronic inflammation is the result of long-term symptoms, there is usually something that needs to be managed to ensure that the body will remain healthy. Chronic inflammation is more likely to develop if someone has any of the following:

- A sensitivity to something, such as food. When the body detects something that it is sensitive to, it usually reacts poorly by triggering inflammation. Hypersensitivity may also lead to allergies.

- Exposure to irritants, such as chemicals, can create chronic inflammation if the exposure is long-term.

- Autoimmune disorders occur when the immune system attempts to attack normal healthy tissues instead of invaders or problematic ones.

- Autoinflammatory diseases that lead to the body's immune system working differently than is normal

- Persistent acute inflammation when the cause is never actually fully treated or recovered from

- Being older and having the body begin to respond to more substances that it is exposed to

- Obesity and the body not having a healthy foundation.

- A diet that is full of unhealthy and inflammatory foods.

- Smoking or ingesting other drugs that are no good for the body to consume.

- Sleep issues lead to the body never resting enough to heal the inflammation that is present within it.

Food and Inflammation

Research has shown that time, and again, inflammation is horrible for the body when it is out of hand and unregulated. Time and again, inflammation will lead to the body struggling or even attempting to attack itself. It is necessary for moderation, but when overactive, it can become dangerous and actually highly disrupt the body. Of course, you probably want to avoid the inflammation that you could be suffering from, and the best way that you can do so is to treat the source.

Food is a very common inflammatory agent that can lead to all sorts of problems. If your body is trying to protect you from the foods that you are consuming, you could run into all sorts of problems just due to the fact that it will be treating the foods as invaders. Inflammation is your body's way of triggering ways to treat itself. It is meant to help you to defend your body and ensure that at the end of the day, you are healthy. In particular, intermittent inflammation can be protective, but when it goes overboard, it will be harmful.

All sorts of highly inflammatory foods trigger the body to respond to them by creating that inflammation. Usually the body is sensitive to the food itself, or to the byproducts of that food being digested, and the end result is that you suffer from inflammation that must be treated somehow. As a result, you end up wanting to find a way that you can manage your symptoms.

Sugars, for example, cause your body to use insulin. Insulin allows your body to take the sugar present in the blood into the cells so that the cells can use the sugars for energy. But, when you have too much sugar in the body at the same time, your body will put sugar into your fat cells, making your fat cells larger and larger. This leads to weight gain and insulin resistance at the same time. The body is not meant to be processing high levels of sugars, and they cause the body all sorts of issues.

Other foods, such as red meats or processed meats, have chemical compounds that are not natural in the human body, and when the body detects them, it then tries to treat them like invaders to protect your body itself. This leads to inflammation when you eat the meats, which over time, can actually lead to heart disease and cancer.

Ultimately, all of these foods will trigger inflammation in different ways, but they are all inflammatory in one way or another. At the end of the day, if you want to be healthy, you will need to find ways that you can treat and manage your inflammation. When you do so, you will realize that you can begin to focus on adding healthier foods just by virtue of understanding how the body breaks them down. Because inflammation can be caused by food, it is important to be aware of how it works and how it breaks down in the body. Likewise, you also want to always know how you can treat inflammation with your own diet as well. By doing so, you should help yourself immensely. Pay attention to your diet, eat well, and you should start to see your diet cleaning itself up so that your inflammation begins to fade as well.

The Consequences of Inflammation

Too much inflammation is horrible for your body. This is why we have anti-inflammatory medication and diets that are meant to help to treat the body's inflammation before it can become bad enough to cause an issue. But, why is it that inflammation is so bad? If it is meant to protect the cells, then how could it possibly be problematic?

There are several consequences of inflammation that are not good at all. Though there are very important benefits to having an immune system that functions and triggers inflammation when it is necessary, it can also cause all sorts of harm that is highly problematic as well.

It is harmful to the guts

Many of the body's immune system cells are all centered around the intestines. Typically, they ignore the bacteria that is supposed to be present in your guts, but for those with autoimmune issues, the body can actually attempt to fight off the bacteria in the gut. As a result, the body's immune cells trigger when they should not, and chronic inflammation is created. This is known as inflammatory bowel disease (IBD) and is an overarching term for several different diseases that lead to diarrhea, ulcers, cramps, and more.

It is harmful to the joints

The joints can also have a horrible effect when exposed to inflammation. In particular, the joints can become highly damaged by the degree of inflammation as it builds up around them. In some cases, arthritis is formed when the body struggles to regulate inflammation around the joints. Those with arthritis of all kinds find that their joints are inflamed and that they cannot move well.

It has been linked to heart disease

Inflammation is also commonly related to heart disease. This is because any part of the body that is damaged is then going to trigger inflammation. This includes the insides of the blood vessels and the heart itself. As fatty plaque is built in the arteries, it triggers chronic inflammation. The plaques then attract white blood cells and grow more and more. They may even cause blood clots that cause a heart attack.

This is even more related to inflammation due to overeating or obesity. Additionally, people who may have a healthy weight but suffer from chronic inflammation in other contexts, such as those with psoriasis, rheumatoid arthritis, or even celiac disease, appear to have higher risks of heart disease despite their weight.

It has been linked to cancer

Additionally, it is also possible that inflammation can be a potential cause of cancer as the body continues to attack certain parts of the body. This could be a major concern for most people as well—after all, no one wants to be diagnosed with cancer.

It can cause problems with sleep

When you have inflammation, you often find that you will be struggling to sleep as well. And, that lack of sleep can also make your inflammation worse as well, creating a sort of double-whammy on your sleep and preventing you from getting that sleep that you will need to treat your body and ensure that you get the rest that you need.

It harms the lungs

When there is inflammation in the respiratory system, it can lead to fluid accumulation, along with the airways narrowing. Together, both of these issues make breathing more difficult than it should be. As a result, the individual may struggle to get the air needed and could need medical intervention to get it. Infections, asthma, and other disease are also linked to this sort of inflammation.

It makes it harder to lose weight

Because inflammation can influence how your body responds to hunger and how your metabolism runs, it can actually cause your body to burn fewer calories when you are trying to lose weight. Additionally, it can also make your body resistant to insulin, which can not only make you more likely to develop diabetes but also stop you from being able to lose the weight that you are trying to fight off.

Inflammation has been linked to mental health issues

In particular, inflammation has been found to potentially be linked to depression. In particular, it has been found that inflammation may be related to depressive symptoms that people would commonly assume are caused by depression, such as lacking appetite, sleeping poorly, and having a bad mood. And it has also been found that people with depression tend to have higher levels of inflammation in their blood at the moment as well, potentially lending credence to this idea that the two are linked.

Chapter 2:
Identifying Inflammatory Foods

If you are ready to start fighting your own inflammation, you have to first know which foods go into your diet and which should be avoided. After all, if only certain foods are responsible for the increase in inflammation, you are going to want to know what they are to protect yourself. If you want to be able to treat yourself well, you will need to know which foods are more likely to cause issues for your body and which will help to alleviate these symptoms.

When you go forward in this book to begin creating the recipes provided, you will be exposed to all sorts of different recipes with all sorts of different ingredients. While you could just take the word of this book for it and trust that the ingredients listed are going to be beneficial to you, it is a good idea for you to understand why these ingredients matter and why they will help you to avoid running into many of the inflammatory-related issues that you could find yourself suffering from. As you learn which ingredients are going to be beneficial and which will be harmful, you can even begin to move beyond the recipes in the book and create your own meals that are going to be beneficial to alleviating your degree of inflammation present in your body. We will first take the time to go over the foods to avoid and then discuss the foods that you should be emphasizing in your diet. From there, we will also take the time to discuss what you can do to ensure that you are getting those good foods in your diet where you want them. This will help you to ensure that at the end of the day, you are getting only the best possible foods and ensuring that you cut that inflammation as much as possible.

Common Inflammatory Foods to Avoid

There are several different foods that are terrible for your health and should be avoided as much as possible. The foods that you are about to see listed out for you are some of the most inflammatory options for you that are not going to be doing you any favors at all. You will want to cut these out as quickly as possible to ensure that at the end of the day, you will be able to maintain your health and help yourself fend off that inflammation.

If you decide that you must have any of these ingredients, however, remember that they should only be present in moderation in your diet. The whole point of this diet isn't to tell you that you can never enjoy a cupcake on a special occasion again—rather, it is to inform you so that you make good, healthy food choices to ensure that you are as healthy as possible. The point is to put the choice back in your hands so you can make the decisions that you want and ensure that the foods that you enjoy are the ones that you really want to keep around.

Sugar

Added sugar might taste great, but it is terrible for the body. It actively triggers the creation of cytokines in the body. Remember, cytokines are those proteins that you are seeking to avoid that tell your body to begin the inflammation process. Because of this effect of adding more inflammation when you consume the added sugars in your diet, it is generally a good idea for you to tackle your inflammation head-on by cutting out the sugars and ensuring that you eat foods that are naturally sweet. Now, you might think that this means that you need to cut out other sweet foods or foods that are filled with natural sugars, but that is not the case. Processed sugars are the problematic ones, especially when they are added in addition to other foods. Signs that there are processed sugars in your food include ingredients such as:

- Fructose

- Galactose

- Glucose

- Lactose

- Maltose

- Sucrose

- Any other names ending in –ose

Refined grains

Like sugars, refined grains are problematic for the body for many of the same reasons. They break down far too rapidly in the body, and the blood sugar swinging is problematic. The foods that you will need to cut out, then, are those that are filled with refined carbs. As a general rule, white flour, bread, and other carbs are going to be the ones to avoid. You want to cut out any of those all-purpose flours and the like—they are problematic for the body and will trigger inflammation in many.

Desserts

Desserts are commonly avoided because they are loaded up with both sugar and refined carbs. They have both of those problematic ingredients, and because of that, they ought to be avoided. They are also usually simply unhealthy due to the caloric intake when they are consumed. If you want to have a sweet treat, the best options use fresh, natural sweeteners as well as whole-wheat products.

Processed meats

Processed meats are usually loaded with a bunch of ingredients that are problematic for you. When you eat foods loaded with trans fats, salts, and other preservatives, your body is not likely to respond well. There is a connection between processed meat consumption and cancer that is undeniable—many cases of colon, esophageal, and lung cancer have been linked to the consumption of processed meats, likely due to the preservation methods used. The most common include types of sausage, bacon, ham, and salami.

Processed seed and vegetable oils

Many common cooking oils with vegetable sources are actually very high in omega-6 fatty acids. While you need these omega-6 acids, you still need to be mindful of the ratio between the omega-3s and omega-6s. Without that ratio balanced out the correct way, you can actually make your inflammation so much worse. Additionally, these oils have been linked to inflammatory diseases such as heart disease and cancer.

Trans fats

Trans-fatty acids, shortened usually to just trans fats, are known to be highly inflammatory. Not only do they cause you to have higher levels of "bad" cholesterol, but they also reduce good cholesterol as well. They are also linked to inflammation, insulin resistance, and obesity, all of which leave you open t potentially suffering from all sorts of other problems. You want to be able to cut out the trans fats if you want to keep yourself healthy, and that means foods such as fast foods, deep-fried foods, baked goods, or anything containing vegetable shortening or partially hydrogenated oil are out.

Alcohol

Alcohol is not only bad for you; it is also inflammatory. High consumption of alcohol is linked to inflammation of the esophagus, larynx, and liver, and it is believed that over time, chronic inflammation from the alcohol can actually begin to cause cancer. All alcohols should either be avoided entirely or drank in moderation to prevent these problems.

Red meats

Many red types of meat have been found to have *Neu5Gc* within them—a compound that is not naturally produced by humans. As a result, the immune system begins to develop anti-Neu5Gc antibodies in response, treating the present as an intruder that needs to be eliminated. These antibodies are then linked to the chronic inflammatory response that is typically meant to be treated with the anti-inflammatory diet in the first place.

Dairy products

Many dairy products trigger all sorts of issues. Milk itself is a common allergen that is linked to IBS, acne, hives, and other inflammatory processes. It is currently estimated that up to 60% of the population actually cannot properly digest milk, leading to all sorts of issues. It is strongly recommended that you avoid all sorts of dairy products, including butter and cheese, if possible. Keep in mind that many other items may have milk ingredients as well that you will need to keep an eye out for in case you are sensitive to them. Thankfully, however, there are many healthier options that you can use that are not inflammatory.

Common Anti-Inflammatory Foods

Of course, if you will be following this diet, you are going to need to know which foods are going to help you the most. If you want to know what the best foods for you to eat on this diet are, you will want to consult this list and everything provided on it to ensure that you know which foods will help you and which will not. These are thirteen foods that are beneficial to consume in your diet to help you alleviate that inflammation. If you are familiar with diets such as the Mediterranean diet, you already know several of these foods and just how healthy they can be in your diet.

Berries

Berries are loaded with all sorts of beneficial aspects that will help you to stay healthy. They are loaded with fiber, minerals, and vitamins that your body needs, and in particular, many of them are also quite high in antioxidants as well. It is that antioxidant power that makes these foods so integral to your diet. In particular, berries have anthocyanins within them that allow you to get that anti-inflammatory effect. This works because your body creates natural killer (NK) cells that are meant to help your body regulate its immune system. In studies, it has been shown that those who consume blueberries on a daily basis actually produce significantly more NK cells than those who do not. Additionally, overweight people who consume strawberries have been found to have lower levels of inflammatory markers that are usually indicative of heart disease.

Grapes

Like berries, grapes are full of anthocyanins. These will allow for that same inflammation-fighting power that berries got. However, beyond just that, they also are loaded with other disease-fighting compounds that will help you to maintain your health and cut the inflammation. One of those is resveratrol, a compound that is believed to have plenty of anti-inflammatory benefits as well.

In a study done on people with heart disease who were consuming grape extract daily, they showed a marked decrease in markers for inflammation, and they also saw an increase of adiponectin—a hormone which is associated with weight gain and cancer when in lower levels.

Broccoli

Broccoli is a cruciferous veggie, along with kale, cauliflower, and brussels sprouts. Cruciferous vegetables are known to be associated with a decreased risk of heart disease and cancer, likely due to the antioxidant content within them. Cruciferous veggies are loaded with antioxidants such as sulforaphane, one that is known to drop the level of cytokines to eliminate the inflammation.

Avocados

Avocados are loaded with all sorts of beneficial vitamins and minerals that are meant to help your body to fend off inflammation, and they are also loaded up with all sorts of antioxidants as well that are good for you. Their nutritional value is what helps them to lower inflammation, especially due to the inclusion of heart-healthy fats. It has been shown that the inclusion of avocado with a hamburger actually showed lower levels of inflammatory markers than was present in people who only ate the burger.

Extra virgin olive oil

One of the primary components of the Mediterranean diet, a well-known anti-inflammatory diet, is extra virgin olive oil. This is one of the healthiest oils that you can get your hands on, and when you choose to consume it, you will be enjoying an oil that tastes not only great but also is full of monounsaturated fats—the healthy fats that help your body to cut its risk of heart disease. EVOO is a potent source of oleocanthal, the antioxidant that is believed to work quite similarly to ibuprofen. Keep in mind that you want to have the least-processed version of oil that you can get, and that means sticking to the extra virgin variant.

Fatty fish

Fatty fish give you a fantastic source of protein while also including the long-chain omega-3 fatty acids known as EPA and DHA, both of which your body needs. These help to reduce inflammation that is commonly associated with metabolic syndrome, kidney and heart diseases, and diabetes. This is because your body processes fatty acids into compounds known as resolvins and protectins, both of which are loaded with anti-inflammatory properties. In particular, you will want to consume fish such as salmon, anchovies, mackerel, herring, or sardines to get the best benefits and enjoy a healthy diet.

Nuts

In particular, both walnuts and almonds are loaded up with all sorts of healthy fats and fiber. They are also low in unhealthy saturated fats as well. As a result, these little foods can actually be a great source of anti-inflammatory power in your diet, especially if you eat them in moderation. Keep in mind that nuts are quite calorie-dense, however, so you will need to be mindful of how you incorporate them into your diet. You must consume them in moderation.

Dark chocolate

Dark chocolate is a great way for you to enjoy that sweet chocolate flavor while still getting the benefits of cutting your risk of inflammation as well. When you enjoy dark chocolate, you get a dose of flavanols that are filled with the anti-inflammatory properties that you are looking for. In particular, it has been found that smokers who enjoy dark chocolate will show a significant improvement in their endothelial function. This means that the lining in their arteries is shown to be functioning better within just two hours of consuming dark chocolate.

Keep in mind that if you are choosing to consume this chocolate, you will need to do so with at least a 70% rating, but higher percentages of cocoa are always better. This will allow you to get those anti-inflammatory benefits that you are looking for. This will be a staple in many of the anti-inflammatory desserts if you do choose to make any.

Tomatoes

Though tomatoes are a part of the nightshade family and that nightshade family may be inflammatory to some, they are also loaded with nutrients that help them to protect your body. In particular, they are loaded with vitamin C, potassium, and the antioxidant known as lycopene. Lycopene is believed to reduce the compounds in your body that may create a higher risk of cancer. And, in drinking tomato juice, it has been found that women with excess weight (but not obesity) actually saw a decrease in inflammatory markers.

Additionally, you will want to ensure that you are constantly pairing your tomatoes with olive oil. Lycopene is best absorbed when it is paired with fat due to the fact that it is a carotenoid. This means that by simply combining your oil and your tomato, you can be sure that you get even more of the inflammation-fighting benefits that you were looking for.

Cherries

When you consume cherries on a regular basis, you are getting both anthocyanins and catechins, both of which will help your body to fend off inflammation. This is essential to you—if you want to cut the inflammation, you want to go for the cherries. In particular, tart cherries are known to have a larger effect, but sweet cherries are still incredibly good for you.

Turmeric

Turmeric is a strong spice that is commonly associated with curry. It gives curry that characteristic scent and color to it and is also highly popular in other Indian dishes. In particular, turmeric is loaded with curcumin, an anti-inflammatory nutrient that is known to reduce inflammation. In particular, turmeric provides you with a method to treat arthritis, diabetes, and more just thanks to its anti-inflammatory powers.

In addition, it is commonly paired with black pepper, thanks to the prevalence of piperine found in pepper. This will show a high decrease in the inflammatory marker CRP found in those suffering from metabolic syndrome.

Green tea

Green tea is commonly touted as one of the healthiest drinks that you can enjoy, and for a good reason. It is known to reduce the risk of heart disease, obesity, cancer, and several other medical conditions, and this is primarily thanks to the antioxidant and anti-inflammatory nature of one of its primary substances. Within green tea, you get high levels of epigallocatechin-3-gallate (ECGC). This is known to reduce inflammation by working on cutting down the levels of cytokines and slow down their production. By inhibiting that production, there is also inhibition of damage to the fatty acids present as well.

Red wine

Though red wine is a form of alcohol, it is also loaded up with resveratrol, which is known to be anti-inflammatory. It is a fantastic option if you are looking for a glass with dinner, but keep in mind that all alcohol should be consumed in moderation. If you want to be able to enjoy the benefits of red wine, you must drink in moderation, and that means only drinking a single glass a few times per week. Too much red wine will be unhealthy and undo the health benefits.

Peppers

Though some people may find that they have problems with peppers, they are also high in both antioxidants and vitamin C, which is known to reduce inflammation. In particular, bell peppers are known to be full of quercetin, while chili peppers are filled up with sinapic and ferulic acids, both of which are believed to reduce inflammation.

Mushrooms

There are thousands of different fungus species out in the world, but only a few of them are actually edible and good for you. Edible mushrooms, however, are incredibly healthy. They are low in calories while also being high in important vitamins and minerals that will keep you healthy. And in addition to that, they are full of phenols and other important antioxidants that will help your body to stay as healthy as possible. One mushroom that excels at this is the lion's mane mushroom—this mushroom is believed to reduce low-grade inflammation related to obesity. However, if you will be adding mushrooms into your diet, remember that they are best served raw as cooking begins to dramatically cut the level of anti-inflammatory compounds present within them.

Avoiding Inflammatory Foods

When you want to start cutting out inflammatory foods, the best thing that you can do is find an appropriate substitute for the various foods that you have to leave behind. For example, you might be letting go of your daily cookie, but you can enjoy a dark chocolate square or a dish made with dark chocolate and other anti-inflammatory ingredients. You might be sensitive to milk, but you could find that you are able to enjoy coconut yogurt instead. These sorts of substitutions are perfect for figuring out how t get those foods that you want into your diet without being unhealthy.

One common substitution that is made is cutting out white carbs. This includes those such as white bread, white flours, and white pasta. Instead, you can replace them with brown varieties that are whole-grain. The whole-grain variants are important because the white carbs will typically spike blood sugar, which is no good for your body when you are attempting to eliminate inflammation. Choosing whole-grain options will help you to ensure that you are healthier just due to the fact that you will be providing yourself with an option that is loaded up in fiber, which will slow down the digestion process, which in turn slows down the way that your body will digest the sugars as well.

Another common change that is made to people's diets is making a point to shift out your butter or other oils for olive oil. Oftentimes, shifting to olive oil works well in most dishes. You can use olive oil on bread, in pasta and rice, and as the primary oil for whatever you are cooking. It might not work so well in baking, but you have several other options as well that will help you to remain as healthy as possible.

It is also strongly recommended that you try to cut ut the added salts on this diet as well. This is because salts are not very good for you—but you can flavor the foods that you are eating with fresh herbs instead. This is a great way for you to ensure that you are getting good foods with ease without causing your body to have any additional inflammation.

Chapter 3:
Adapting the Anti-Inflammatory Diet and Lifestyle

If you are ready to start cutting out the inflammation in your body by changing your diet, then one of the best starting points is by adapting the anti-inflammatory diet and lifestyle to ensure that you are as healthy as possible. Ultimately, your diet is meant to be all-encompassing—you have to not only change the foods that you consume but also your habits to ensure that at the end of the day, you make choices that are effective and beneficial to you. This will help you to figure out precisely what you will want to enjoy and how you will want to spend your day.

Within this chapter, we have plenty of considerations to make to ensure that you get the fullest extent of all of the information that you are going to need to know. We will first address what the anti-inflammatory diet is and then follow up with understanding the benefits of the anti-inflammatory diet. We will go over how you can follow this diet to get the right benefits, as well as look at several different examples of diets that could be considered anti-inflammatory with how they work. Ultimately, the right diet for you will be highly dependent upon your preferences and the type of inflammation that you are suffering from. When you address this the right way, you will start to see that you can make very real changes that are significant enough to get you the benefits that you are looking for.

What Is the Anti-Inflammatory Diet?

Anti-inflammatory dieting is more than just sticking to one specific diet. It is actually meant to help you to get that systemic anti-inflammatory effect that you are looking for, and you can do this by adopting any type of anti-inflammatory diet. That's right—there is no one anti-inflammatory diet—the term refers to any diet that is naturally anti-inflammatory in nature or is designed to aid in the alleviation of inflammation as well. There are many different options, but remember this—you are looking for a reduction in inflammation right now. This diet, though it is healthier and may lend itself well to weight loss, is not actually meant to focus on the loss of weight in general. It is all about ensuring that your meals are healthy, well-rounded, and beneficial to you to ensure that you are getting the foods that you will need when you need them. By following this diet, you will find yourself getting all sorts of those benefits without much work at all.

These diets are known to help you fend off inflammation in ways that are highly beneficial to you. Typically, these diets are high in fruits and veggies as the primary source of nutrition for you. And they will also emphasize healthy fats, whole grains, lean protein, and spices over salts. Additionally, it recommends that there is a limit on processed food, alcohol, or red meats.

Keep in mind that there are several different options that will work for you. However, because this diet will focus on plant-based foods, it will also be high in antioxidants. The antioxidants that you consume then allow your body to work to fend off free radicals. When you eat certain inflammatory foods, you are getting that inflammation due to the consumption of foods that will create free radicals. As the free radicals spread throughout the body, they can create stress and inflammation. These free radicals are also natural byproducts of certain processes of the body, such as its digestion of food. However, the free radicals are not good for you—they create damage to the cells, and that then increases your risk of inflammation.

However, when you start utilizing the antioxidant-rich diets that are touted as an anti-inflammatory, you start cutting down those free radicals. Antioxidants actually work to remove free radicals from the body to provide it with the chance to begin to heal.

Benefits of the Anti-Inflammatory Diet

As you begin to eat healthier foods, you start to get all sorts of benefits as well. Doctors around the world recommend that everyone should follow an anti-inflammatory diet—they are highly healthy and beneficial to our general health and wellness as well. Some of the best benefits of this diet include the following:

- **Seeing an improvement in autoimmune and inflammatory disorders:** Because many autoimmune disorders are directly linked to inflammatory issues, it becomes the case that many of them actually begin to be alleviated when you make it a point to consume this diet. Many different ones, such as arthritis, inflammatory bowel syndrome, and lupus, have all been found to be managed well with diet. This means that by taking control of your diet, you should also start to see benefits in how you feel.

- **Decreasing the risk for several diseases and disorders:** Because this diet will have you primarily consuming foods that are healthy for you and are loaded with vitamins and minerals that are good for you, you will start to see the risk of you developing several different diseases, and disorders actually decrease as well. In particular, you could see a lowered risk of obesity, depression, heart disease, cancer, and even diabetes.

- **Reduced levels of inflammatory markers:** Your blood can tell a lot about you, and that includes the level of inflammation found in your body. When you consume this diet, you will lower the markers for inflammation that are present within the body. This is your testament to the fact that this diet is working.

- **Your blood sugar, cholesterol, and triglyceride levels improve:** This diet will also allow your blood to be healthier as well. Your blood sugar will be stable and regulate itself better. Your cholesterol and triglyceride levels will also improve as well during your time consuming this diet. This means that you are getting a healthier heart.

- **Your energy and mood will improve:** You will also see that there is a marked improvement in your mood and energy levels as well. This is directly related to the fact that this diet will help you to better manage your blood sugar. As your blood sugar levels are better managed, you realize that your energy levels also stabilize as well. This is perfect for you and will help you to begin to get that effect that you are looking for.

Who Should Follow This Diet?

If you are wondering if you should get started with diet, you probably have some questions about who is going to be getting the most benefit from doing so. Ultimately, just about anyone would benefit from this diet—just about anyone would find that they have inflammation that could be cut out, and even if they do not currently have inflammation concerns, the truth is that these diets are so healthy that most people would benefit anyway just due to the increase in healthier foods and the reduction of foods that are objectively unhealthy as well.

However, there are several different inflammatory diseases that people may suffer from who would benefit dramatically from getting these benefits brought into their own lives as well. If you are someone who suffers from the following conditions, you might find yourself benefitting from this diet:

- asthma

- colitis

- Crohn's disease

- eosinophilic esophagitis

- Hashimoto's thyroiditis

- rheumatoid arthritis

- inflammatory bowel disease

- lupus

- metabolic syndrome

- psoriasis

Because all of these are believed to have something to do with inflammation, the anti-inflammatory diet options may then begin to treat the problems. This means that by learning to choose your diet well and eating foods that are highly healthy for you, you can start to get all sorts of benefits for yourself as well.

The Mediterranean Diet

One of the most common anti-inflammatory options that people follow when they are working to lose weight is the Mediterranean diet. This diet is based upon the traditional foods that were found in the Mediterranean countries, such as

Greece and Italy, in the 1960s. During the research, it was found that the people in these countries were notably healthier than those found in the United States. They also were found to have a much lower risk of many different diseases as well. Studies showed that these people eating this diet were actually found to have a reduction in symptoms that were commonly associated with heart attacks, type 2 diabetes, strokes, and more. They also lived longer as well.

This diet is all about living as if you were part of that particular demographic. It involves cutting out most red meat and processed foods and instead emphasizing local, farm-fresh foods that you can get in season in your local area. It emphasizes a higher level of plant-based foods while recommending that dairy be eaten in moderation, and red meat should rarely be consumed at all. Beyond that, it strongly recommends that sugary drinks, added sugars, processed foods, and refined foods should be avoided entirely to prevent the body from being unhealthy.

Additionally, this diet emphasizes exercise regularly as a part of it, as well as eating with loved ones or friends at every meal. You are meant to nourish your mind, body, and heart all in one go, enjoying your meals and the company that you keep. This diet has allowed many people to get healthier and is associated as well with the fact that it is highly anti-inflammatory. It naturally drops the rate of inflammation that is found in the body, as can be seen in recognizing the improvement in heart health. This is, by far, one of the most popular options that you have when it comes to following an anti-inflammatory diet.

The DASH Diet

In response to the epidemic of high blood pressure throughout the United States, the National Heart, Lung, and Blood

Institute created the DASH diet. This is the Dietary Approaches to Stop Hypertension (DASH) diet, and it was traditionally recommended for those suffering from high blood pressure. However, it is also good for other people to consume as well because it does emphasize getting healthy foods to provide all of the nutrients that you are looking for from other sources.

This diet is all about getting in higher levels of your nutrients that you need to lower blood pressure, such as potassium, calcium, and protein, while also bulking up on the fiber as well. This plan works toward getting these nutrients into the diet by enjoying fruits, vegetables, and healthy sources of lean protein. Additionally, grains should always be whole, and the diary should be low-fat. Like the Mediterranean diet, this diet recommends a reduction of red meat, sugary foods, and fatty foods while also pushing for a reduction in salt as well.

This diet recommends a spread of foods with the following servings:

- Fat-free or low-fat milk products: 2-3 servings per day

- Fats and oils: 2-3 servings per day

- Fruits: 4-5 servings per day

- Grains: 6-8 servings per day

- Lean meats, poultry, and fish: 6 or fewer servings per day

- Max sodium limit: 2,300 milligrams per day

- Nuts, seeds, and legumes: 3-5 per week

- Sweets and added sugars: 5 or less per week

- Vegetables: 4-5 servings per day

The Low FODMAP Diet

The low FODMAP diet is really only for those who find themselves suffering from irritable bowel syndrome. It is believed that IBS is caused due to a problem with inflammation linked to the diet. It points at FODMAPs—foods that are full of short-chain carbs that are difficult for the body to digest. This diet is meant to aid in eliminating the symptoms of IBS by removing those short-chain carbs in hopes of allowing the body to heal. It is meant to provide the body with the option to get better without much struggle. However, that alone is difficult because FODMAPs are healthy for most people—it is only those suffering from IBS that appear to be sensitive to them.

FODMAPs are fermentable oligosaccharides, disaccharides, monosaccharides, and polyols. Together, this creates the FODMAP group. These are foods that your body naturally needs, but when you are sensitive to them for any reason, they will create the inflammation that causes the symptoms that you are trying to eliminate. For this reason, you will be working on cutting them out. FODMAPs are supposed to feed the healthy bacteria in the guts, but remember—when you have inflammation in the body, it could attack those healthy bacteria and create an unhealthy imbalance that you need to eliminate.

This diet is really only suitable for those diagnosed with IBS, and anyone else may find themselves struggling with it. However, this is another common anti-inflammatory diet that deserves to be acknowledged as well.

The Low-Carb Diet

Because it is the case that many processed carbs and sugars are highly inflammatory, most low-carb diets are naturally anti-inflammatory as well. These are diets that would restrict carbs found in pastas, bread, and other processed foods. Instead of going for those foods that are high in carbs, you would instead emphasize healthy proteins, fats, and veggies. This diet is great for weight loss but is also typically seen as a good low-inflammation diet as well, thanks to how it works.

The Autoimmune Paleo Diet

Another common anti-inflammatory diet is the autoimmune paleo diet. This diet cuts out foods such as added sugars, legumes, dairy, grains, and refined oils. It is meant to create a situation in which you are able to consume primarily natural foods that our ancestors would have eaten. It is meant to focus on the diet that our ancient hunter-gatherer ancestors would have had access to before the invention of farming.

This diet is shown to be anti-inflammatory primarily just due to the fact that you will be cutting out foods that are traditionally considered inflammatory. You will be removing basically all processed foods from your diet, meaning that foods such as cookies, chips, and sodas will be eliminated. Additionally, dairy, grains, and the like are already commonly associated with the issues commonly associated with inflammation. This diet should provide those anti-inflammatory benefits in theory, and you will find several paleo diet recipes throughout this book as well. Be mindful, however, that if you choose to follow the paleo diet, you will need to be mindful of your nutritional intake to ensure that you avoid any deficiency.

The Vegetarian Diet

The vegetarian diet is commonly suggested as well if you were to ask for help coming up with an anti-inflammatory diet for yourself as well. This diet is primarily plant-based and will allow you to cut out many of the inflammation-causing meats that could cause issues. Again, thanks to the fact that plants and plant-based foods are rich in antioxidants, you will find that this diet is fantastic for helping you to cut down on your inflammation levels.

Ultimately, this is a diet that will require you to cut out protein from animal sources entirely. This means that you will have to be careful with how you take care of yourself. You must ensure that you are meeting your nutritional value and will have to take up several protein sources from plants instead.

Choosing the Right Diet for You

When it comes to knowing the right kind of diet for you, you will need to consider what you need, what you want, and what you prefer. This is important here—after all, many of these diet options require you to cut out various sources of food. However, one thing is constant across them all—they all remove the junky foods or red meats that are recognized as highly inflammatory. No matter which of these you choose to follow, you will start getting all sorts of anti-inflammatory benefits.

As you read through this book, you will be getting anti-inflammatory recipes from all of these different diets. Some will be vegetarian or vegan. Others will follow the autoimmune paleo diet. Others still will draw from the Mediterranean diet. You will get all sorts of benefits from these different sources, and that will help you to ensure that you are as healthy as possible. Choosing out the diet that is right for you will be highly personal and depend entirely on what it is that you want out of them. Consider the restrictions for each of the listed anti-inflammatory diets, and then pick the one for you!

Chapter 4:
Healing Your Body With the Anti-Inflammatory Diet

One of the most important reasons that people use the anti-inflammatory diet is because they want to heal their bodies. They want to help their bodies to begin to recover, to soothe the irritation and inflammation that is caused by their diets. When you consider what it is that you can do for yourself just by feeding yourself, you start to get some huge benefits. You will be able to figure out what you can do to provide yourself with those added benefits. When it comes time to heal yourself, making sure that you eat the right foods is a great way to do so. Healing your body matters, after all.

When you work on your diet, you help yourself to be a healthier person. You work to provide yourself with healthier, nourishing foods so that you can heal. You are trying to prevent those inflammatory processes from occurring because you want to also provide your body chances to heal. That means that the inflammation has to have the chance to subside without being triggered again and again. When you follow up with the anti-inflammatory diet, you should find that your body does recover slowly.

Of course, this will take time to actually make it happen. For this reason, those who wish to heal are recommended to take at least 30 days to eliminate the inflammatory foods from their diets. It is highly recommended to allow your body the chance to get rid of the underlying inflammation so that you can be successful and so that you can heal. When you do that, you can usually work with yourself to be happier and healthier.

Within this chapter, we have a few important goals that you are going to need to achieve if you want your own success. If you want to truly get the benefits of the autoimmune diet so that you can begin to heal yourself, you will need to follow along here. You must first consider the elimination phase of this diet, which we will go over shortly. You must also pay attention to how anti-inflammatory foods encourage your body to heal in the first place, addressing how it is that antioxidants benefit the body. From there, we will also go over everything that you will need to know to ensure that you are healthier. We will finally address how it is that this diet heals your body and allows you to do better. At the end of it all, you should have a better understanding and appreciation for how powerful this diet is.

So, no matter why you struggle with your inflammation, and no matter why you want to overcome the inflammation in the first place, this diet is here to help you. This diet is going to teach you everything that you will need to know and do if you want to be successful in eliminating it. We have the ability to heal our bodies and soothe the inflammation where it begins.

The truth is, with the power of plant-based foods and those that follow the Mediterranean diet, we can begin to soothe that inflammation. We can work to prevent it from harming us further. We can stop the processes that hurt us so that we will be able to recover successfully. You will be able to harness this power if you pay close attention to the foods that you eat and why you eat them. When you start being more mindful about your diet, it will get better. When you are more mindful about why you consume the foods that you do, you discover that you can be healthier. All you needed to do was change how you did things. Before you know it, you will be as healthy as you want to be, and that is highly important.

The Elimination Phase of the Anti-Inflammatory Diet

When you follow an anti-inflammatory diet, most of the time, you take the time to follow what is known as the auto-immune protocol. This is a diet plan that is intended to discover the source of inflammation to then ensure that your diet that you consume is going to avoid those triggers. Think of this as sort of your body's way to figure out which things will hurt it and which will actually be beneficial to you. When you go out of your way to figure out the foods that will work for you, you get to create a custom-made diet that you know is going to provide you with all of those key benefits that you will need.

The elimination phase, then, requires you to cut out the most common inflammatory foods in your diet. It requires you to change up how you are eating so that you can be certain that you are on the right track toward healing. It works to give your guts that time without the inflammatory foods that cause you problems. As your guts are not being inundated with foods that they respond to with inflammation, they get the chance to heal. As they heal, they begin to do better.

This phase can be one of the most frustrating for those following the anti-inflammatory diet. Because it will require you to eliminate so many different foods, you might think that it is not worth it, especially if you don't get results immediately. However, remember that healing is a process. Remember that healing will take time and energy, and that means that you will have to actually be patient. The results that you get will usually be worth it.

After you have eliminated all of those foods from your diet, and then gave yourself at least a month, or preferably up to six weeks, for your body to heal, you can then start adding the foods right back in, one by one. You can start adding in those foods that are considered more inflammatory. The idea here is that as you slowly reintroduce foods into your diet, you will start eliminating foods as being problematic for you. While some foods are simply inflammatory for most people, others may be tolerable for you and you would not know that they are tolerable until you get that added boost from those around you. Over time, you should start to see that you can eat a more varied diet and that you can and will be able to enjoy foods that you might have thought initially would be a problem.

How Anti-Inflammatory Foods Soothe Your Body

When you follow any number of the anti-inflammatory diets that you have around you, you can find yourself actually getting great benefits. You should start to see that ultimately, the reason that you are struggling the way that you are is actually because of the food that you eat. But, when you start eating better with the foods emphasized in this diet plan or in diets similar to it, the result is that you get better simply because you wind up cutting out the bad foods while also introducing foods full of antioxidants.

Antioxidants, as we have briefly touched upon, reduce the levels of free radicals in your body. Antioxidants, in protecting your body from all of these free radicals, actually then protect your heart and other parts of your body. There are many, many different types of antioxidants, but the vast majority of them appear in plant-based foods. They will help to repair your body and encourage your body to heal, little by little.

Additionally, however, anti-inflammatory foods are loaded with fiber while also typically being lower in fat as well. This allows the body to better balance itself out. When you are loading yourself up on fiber-rich food, you are keeping your blood sugar levels more stable, and doing so actually betters your health. Fiber also helps your body thanks to the fact that it has lower energy density than other foods, and that allows you to lose weight. Those who eat higher levels of fiber-rich food tend to also have lower body weight. As you lose weight and maintain a healthy one, your body actually heals from inflammation better. This is because obesity is known to be inflammation-inducing in the first place. If you want to reduce the amount of inflammation, you can do so, and you will see great benefits as a result.

Studies have also shown that those with higher levels of fiber in their diet tend to have lower levels of C-reactive protein (CRP) in their blood. CRP is known to be a marker for inflammation that is specifically linked to autoimmune disorders. This is exactly why this diet will focus so heavily on fruits and vegetables. In fact, you may even see a greater effect if you were to entirely cut out animal-based protein sources and focused on a vegetarian or vegan version of this diet. As you read through this book, you will see that there are several recipes that are meant to emphasize vegetarian and vegan options. That is not to say that you cannot enjoy the occasional piece of fish or chicken, and you will see recipes that recommend both, but take a page out of the Mediterranean diet's book and recognize that one of the best things you can do for your health is to limit the amount of animal-sourced foods you eat.

The Effect of Avoiding Inflammatory Irritants from Your Diet

The unfortunate reality is that the standard American diet is pro-inflammatory. This means that the standard diet that most Americans eat is going to cause you those problems with inflammation, most of which would stem from the fact that you are eating foods that are highly processed. When you consume these foods, you end up unintentionally causing your body to become even more inflamed than it was before. When you start avoiding these foods, however, you do your body a big favor. By cutting those foods out of your diet entirely, you can actually help your body to begin healing.

Avoiding irritants gives your body that time to heal. It is believed that many autoimmune conditions occur because there is a problem with the bacteria within the gut. Due to the imbalance in the gut biome, the individual is more likely to suffer from toxins, viruses, or even just byproducts of the food being digested, to breach through the gut wall. As a result, there are all sorts of various toxins or foreign material floating around in the body. As a result, inflammation occurs. The inflammation happens because the body is trying to reduce the prevalence of these foreign bodies. And, sometimes, the body's immune response ends up being too strong, leading to the autoimmune symptoms in the first place. The end result, according to this theory, is the autoimmune disease that you are trying to avoid.

Another theory states that the composition of the gut biome may actually lead to inflammation in the body if it is not balanced. An unhealthy gut can wreak havoc on just about every part of the body, and if they cause inflammation, then healing the gut biome by fixing the diet would also help alleviate that inflammation as well.

It has also been found that inflammation actually changes how the gut wall functions. When you are allergic to something and consume it, you can actually see the gut wall become more porous as a result. This could further create that connection between problems with the gut and the creation of autoimmune diseases. You could simply be sensitive to inflammatory foods, and as a result, you realize that you cannot consume those foods without causing issues.

Essentially, avoiding inflammatory foods allows you to avoid all of the aforementioned problems with inflammation. When the problem with your symptoms is due to the food that you consume, cutting those foods out of your diet, in theory, would then heal your body entirely.

Healing Your Body

If you have ever had a serious injury or been recovering from surgery, you were probably told to eat certain foods. The foods recommended are typically highly nutritious, and this is for a good reason. Those highly nutritious foods tend to be loaded up with antioxidants, and those antioxidants are typically incredibly effective at providing you with those healing boosts that you are going to need. When you enjoy the foods on this diet, you provide your body with the antioxidants needed to prevent a buildup of reactive oxygen species, which is created when the cells break down. The breakdown of cells could be due to injury or due to inflammation in parts of the body.

When you are ready to heal your body, there are certain parts of the foods that will help you to heal. If you want the best anti-inflammatory effect, you will want to implement the following nutrients to your own diet:

- **Antioxidants:** These are found primarily in vitamins A, C, and E, and they help to mitigate oxidative stress that can be inflammatory.

- **Anthocyanins:** These are found in foods that are primarily purple, blue, or red, and they work to reduce down inflammation in the body.

- **Vitamin D:** This is in fatty fish, eggs, cheese, or foods fortified with vitamin D, and this also helps you to reduce inflammation levels.

- **Nitric oxide and nitrates:** These are found in leafy greens, beets, and celery, and they work to help increase blood flow in order to reduce inflammation.

- **Omega 3 fatty acids:** This is found in fatty fish and certain seeds and nuts, and it is known to reduce levels of inflammation.

When you see foods that are recognized for their prowess at cutting down inflammation levels, usually, those levels are reduced because of the aforementioned categories of nutrients.

Chapter 5:
How to Meal Plan

Now, being able to follow along with this diet can be difficult. It can be tough for you to follow along with how you can meal plan, but this chapter is here to help. One of the biggest problems that people tend to run into when it comes to dieting is feeling like they don't know what they are doing or deciding that they are too tired to figure out a diet-friendly option for themselves. They tell themselves that sticking to their diet is simply too much effort, so they skip it.

The truth is, however, that meal planning isn't difficult. It can actually be highly streamlined with a little process known as meal planning. When you meal plan, you set everything up, so the mental power of coming up with what you will make for dinner after a long day is no longer a problem for you. This will help you to ensure that you stick to your diet simply because you will already know what to expect and know what you will make at all times.

What Is Meal Planning?

Meal planning might seem like it is difficult. It might seem like it is nearly impossible in many situations. How can you possibly know what you want to eat for dinner a week in advance? But, knowing what you are going to eat is actually a huge benefit—when you know what's for dinner, you don't have to stop yourself to figure out what you should be eating. When you meal plan accordingly, you should be able to zoom through the understanding of what you need and why.

Meal planning is essentially telling yourself that you will only ask yourself what's for breakfast, lunch, or dinner just once a week. When you have that question just once instead of every single day, it becomes easier to not only stick to a diet but also to figure out what you need to purchase. When you follow your meal plan, you should be able to change your diet with ease, and you should discover whether or not you are able to make those big changes in your life. The purpose of meal planning is to give you that structure that you will need to stick to your diet. It will give you the power that you will need to make those good choices.

How to Meal Plan

Meal planning is incredibly simple. All you will have to do is follow three simple steps. These steps are:

1. Select your meals and recipes

2. Shop for all ingredients that you will need

3. Prepare your ingredients

Ideally, you would start on a Friday (or whatever day goes into your two days off from work) so that you can follow along easily. Starting by selecting your meals on Friday night. This will allow you to start filling out your meal plans for the week. You will see an example of this at the end of the book. You want to figure out what you intend to eat for the week. This will help you to figure out exactly what you are going to need to purchase to ensure that you have all of your ingredients.

When you work on putting together your meal plan, make sure that you also pay attention to the schedule that you have. You want to ensure that you are providing yourself with foods that you know are going to actually line up with the real-time responsibilities that you have. This means that you should not be creating those meals that are going to be difficult to cook on days when you are stretched thin for time. Making sure that meals line up with the severity of the time that you have available to you is important, and that means making sure that your schedules check out. When you ensure that you have meals that will feasibly fit into your schedule, you know that you are taking the time to do what is going to work for you. This makes your meal plan more realistic and grants you that freedom. You won't feel like you are too pressed for time to create that big meal when you know that you schedule it on a day that you are not very busy.

Saturday morning, you can do your shopping. Remember that you should be at the grocery store with a plan to follow your diet strictly. You want to provide yourself with just the foods that you know are going to be nutritious and healthy for you. When you keep yourself on track with your shopping list, you will make sure that your kitchen is well stocked with all of the nutritious foods that you know that you can enjoy. This will protect you and ensure that you are only consuming foods that are going to be good for you.

Then, Sunday, you can do any prep that needs to be done. If you need to take care of cutting up ingredients, so they are ready for you, you can do that. If you are preparing meat for the week, you can do that as well. Ultimately, you are trying to provide yourself with everything that you can do to keep your schedule. You might be surprised to realize that, really, you can cut up your ingredients ahead of time. Do you need a whole bunch of chopped veggies for your dinner? You can chop them all Sunday morning and then keep them in the fridge until they are needed. This will help you to save time when you might need that extra time, and will also help you greatly.

Of course, not all ingredients can be prepped so far in advance. You might not want to chop up tomatoes on Sunday to use on Friday, but you certainly can make sure that you are using other veggies that you will keep so you can be more informed about your diet ad ensure that you are only consuming the best. If you want to figure out what you will need to do to keep yourself fed and happy, you want to pay close attention to the foods that you choose and also make it easier than ever to grab the foods that you will be enjoying and using.

Meal Planning Tips and Tricks

When you're ready to start meal planning, you might feel a bit overwhelmed at everything. It can be tough to figure out what you will need to do and how you should be doing it. But, if you know what you are doing, you can figure out how best you can stick to your meal plan. Not only will you give your guts the chance to heal by doing so, but you will also get to enjoy the foods. Consider these choices that you can make for yourself.

Make a COMPLETE menu

When you are meal planning, it can help to make sure that you have a complete menu. This means that you should schedule your breakfast, lunch, dinner, and snacks for each day of the week. This helps you to understand what you will need to buy when you are shopping. You will be certain that you have the right amounts of everything, which also helps you to lower food costs and also prevent waste at the same time.

Plan around foods that are on sale

When you plan to make a menu for the week, make sure that you consider foods that are on sale for the week. Always check out your local ads before you begin meal planning. If you notice that one or two protein sources are particularly on sale, you will be able to plan your meals around that instead.

Plan meatless at least once a week

Meat is expensive, time-consuming to prepare, and also inflammatory. When at all possible, you should plan a few meatless meals per week to provide yourself with the foods that you are enjoying. When you are considering the meals that you will eat for the week, consider making it a point to have at least one meal per week that is vegetarian or vegan. When you do this, you will provide yourself with plenty of foods that will help you. This is essential to alleviating your inflammation and will be a great way to help yourself.

Avoid recipes that have special ingredients

When you are meal planning, avoid any meals that will require you to use special ingredients. For example, if you are going to be making use of foods that are special or specific to just one meal, you are going to spend more money. What are you going to do with leftover leek if only one meal on your meal plan uses them? What are you going to do with a big bottle of miso paste if only one meal will require it? You end up wasting extra food that could have been better used. This is why it is so essential to meal plan around the same ingredients for the week—it lowers your overall cost.

Look seasonal

Ultimately, the fresher the ingredients, the better they are because the nutritional content is able to be maintained. When food is harvested, it starts to degrade, and that means that you will be losing nutrients. Studies have shown that most products actually lose around 30% of their nutritional content within three days of harvest, and it all goes downhill from there. When you go over everything, you should be able to find those seasonal foods that are going to benefit you. You just want to figure out what it is at the moment. You want to make sure that you eat those local foods, which are fresher and usually harvested more recently.

Make extra and plan to eat leftovers

You should also make it a point to make extras of meals where you can. Typically, it is cheaper to double a batch of food that you are cooking than it is to cook a second meal because you will have some of the ingredients already, and buying one larger batch is usually easier than buying the ingredients for several meals. If you wanted to, you could also save yourself time by making a large batch and then using the rest of the leftovers for your lunches to reheat at work. These ways allow you to save time and money simply by making extra food. You should also make sure that there is a day each week that you just use leftovers. That leftover day could also become takeout day if you and your family enjoy getting food from restaurants as well.

Meal plan to your taste

Finally, consider what happens if you meal plan to your specific taste. Many diets can be frustrating—they have foods that you might not actually care to eat. They could also be loaded up with all sorts of foods that you don't like. This can make it difficult to stick to your diet. If you don't like the foods that you are eating, you are going to struggle to stick to the diet, so by making sure that your meal plan to the taste you have, you will be more successful. The good thing about this diet is that it is loaded up with ingredients, and you are able to figure out the right foods for you. When you do this the right way, you can keep yourself on track. You will enjoy every moment on your diet because you will be eating foods that you enjoy.

Chapter 6:
Choosing Foods for Your Shopping List

Of course, when you are getting ready to diet, you will also need to choose the right kinds of foods to put on your shopping list. You will need to ensure that you plan how you should eat and why you should enjoy the foods that you do. This will help you to succeed on this diet so you can feel your body begin to heal. Having a grocery list that is well-planned helps you to stick to a budget, streamlines shopping, and also helps you to figure out how you can manage your diet well. Ultimately, the more that you do this, the easier it will get. But, consider the following information to help you stick to your budget and your diet. Your wallet and your body will thank you!

Grocery Shopping on a Budget

Food is one of the most expensive parts of just about anyone's budget. It is incredibly important to know how you can budget and shop to eat well, but once you learn to do so, you will be able to thrive. Consider these points to keep your budget under control while still shopping well.

- **Learn the pricing:** When you are shopping, pay attention to the various stores and what they charge for all of the items that you buy regularly. You may be surprised to find that spreading out where you do your shopping can actually benefit you. You might be able to change up your shopping plans to pocket a decent amount of the money on hand to help yourself manage to spend.

- **Shop the exteriors of the stores:** When you go through the grocery store, you should focus on shopping the exterior of the shop. This means that you will be looking for whole foods. These are typically far cheaper than buying the processed version, and you only have a bit more work to do. You might find that you need to do a bit more cutting of your items, or you might have to choose to prepare your seasonings from scratch, but you will be able to save some money.

- **Learn which store brands are good:** This will be largely to taste, but there are several foods that are perfectly fine when you buy generic. When you do this, you will actually be able to pick out foods that are cheaper but still just as good.

- **Buy in bulk and reuse ingredients:** One of the reasons it is a good idea to plan meals around similar ingredients every time is because when you do, you can buy larger quantities. If you know that you are going to use chicken and bell peppers to make fajitas, try planning out a second meal that also uses chicken and bell peppers. You will usually save more money.

Planning Ahead

Of course, you must also meal plan. We've discussed this already. If you know what meals that you are going to make for the week, make sure that you write them all down. Take the time to record those ingredients, so you know that you got them all when you do go shopping. The more that you can record down, the better you will do. Choosing out the right ingredients will help you to successfully get through everything that you need. To better understand this step, return to the chapter on meal planning and use the tips there. You will discover that you can actually make great progress.

Know What You Currently Have in Stock

Of course, when you are making your grocery list, you should also consider going through what you currently have. You want to make sure that you've got the right tools on hand. Sometimes, you might already have several ingredients as well. This is an important point to consider as well—double-check the foods that you currently have so you can then start using what you do have on hand. When you use up ingredients that you already have, such as using rice when you already have it, you get to cut down on the foods that you have to buy. This is where having a well-stocked pantry can be great for you. When you have that pantry built up, you can then purchase just what you need, and that will help you to save money as well. After all, meal planning and budgeting don't need to be impossible. You can usually make this work with ease. Choosing out the right foods will help you immensely. It will ensure that you always have everything that you will need on hand, meaning that sticking to your diet is easier.

Buy Exactly What You Need

Finally, your meal plan should be complete. You should have all of your breakfasts, lunches, dinners, and snacks recorded, and that is something that you will be able to use to manage your money. You will be able to buy only the ingredients that you will need, and by doing so, you can keep track of your diet better. You will manage both your diet and your budget, and that will help you to keep yourself on track.

Chapter 7:
Anti-Inflammatory Breakfasts

Breakfasts are incredibly important, whether you are trying to cut out inflammatory foods or not. By starting your day off on the right foot with these anti-inflammatory breakfasts, you should see that this diet is going to provide you with the much-needed energy that you will need to get through everything on your schedule. Of course, some of these breakfasts will be freshly made, while others will be make-ahead recipes that you can take with you for ease on those busy days when you have too much going on to get started on your own. Choose out your favorite recipes and give them a try—they will be highly enjoyable.

<u>Avocado and Kale Omelet</u>

Ingredients:

- Avocado (a quarter of one, sliced)

- Crushed red pepper

- Eggs (2)

- Fresh cilantro (1 Tbsp., chopped)

- Kale (1 c., chopped)

- Lime juice (1 Tbsp.)

- Milk (1 tsp)

- Olive oil (2 tsp)

- Salt

- Unsalted sunflower seeds (1 tsp)

Instructions:

1. Whip the milk, eggs, and salt. Heat up a teaspoon of your oil in a skillet over medium heat. Pour in the eggs and cook until the bottom has set, but the middle is still runny. Flip the omelet, cooking for a few more seconds, then move to a serving plate.

2. In a bowl, toss the kale with the remaining oil, cilantro, lime juice, sunflower seeds, salt, and crushed red pepper. Top your omelet with the salad and garnish with the avocado slices. Serve.

<u>*Turmeric Scrambled Eggs*</u>

Ingredients:

- Cumin (quarter tsp)

- Eggs (8)

- Salt and pepper

- Turmeric powder (1 tsp)

- Unsweetened almond milk (half c.)

Instructions:

1. Prepare your oven by heating it up to 350° F. Get a casserole dish and lightly grease it.

2. Whip your eggs, turmeric, milk, pepper, and salt together. Pour the eggs into the casserole dish and move the casserole into the oven. Bake for ten minutes and then remove from heat. Stir the eggs to give them a good scramble and place them back in the oven.

3. Bake for an additional eight minutes and then remove from heat. Stir the eggs one last time and begin serving.

Veggie Breakfast Muffins

Ingredients:

- Alcohol-free vanilla extract (1 tsp)

- Apple cider vinegar (1 Tbsp.)

- Avocado oil (3 Tbsp.)

- Baking soda (1 tsp)

- Carrot (two-thirds c., shredded)

- Cinnamon (2 tsp)

- Coconut flour (3 Tbsp.)

- Dried fruit (quarter c., your pick)

- Gala apple (1, finely chopped)

- Ginger (1 tsp)

- Green plantains (2, chopped)

- Parsnip (two-thirds c., shredded)

- Pumpkin puree (half c.)

- Raisins (quarter c.)

- Sea salt (quarter tsp)

Instructions:

1. In order to have the muffins bake well, set your oven's temperature to 375° F. Setup a muffin pan or two by greasing lightly with oil or cooking spray. Alternatively, use muffin pan liners.

2. Grab your plantains, pumpkin puree, avocado oil, apple cider vinegar, and vanilla extract, and place them in a blender or food processor. Pulse until the mixture is smooth.

3. Combine all the ingredients into a large bowl and mix thoroughly.

4. Pour in the batter into the muffin pans, making sure not to fill the spaces to the top. You want some space for the muffins to fluff into and expand.

5. Place the muffin pan(s) into the oven and bake for 30 minutes.

6. Check to make sure your muffins have baked through and remove them from the oven. Allow them to cool for 15 minutes before removing them from the muffin pan. Set them on a wire rack and allow them to cool before plating and serving.

Instant Pot Cinnamon Porridge

Ingredients:

- Chia seeds (1 Tbsp.)

- Cinnamon (half tsp)

- Coconut milk (half c.)

- Maple syrup to sweeten

- Powdered ginger (1 tsp)

- Roasted sunflower seeds (3 Tbsp.)

- Sea salt (a dash)

- Squash (1 c., chopped and pre-cooked)

- Turmeric powder (just a dash)

- Unsweetened shredded coconut (2 Tbsp.)

Instructions:

1. Begin by taking all the dry ingredients and putting them into a blender or grinder. Process the mixture into a fine powder. Once done, mix with the coconut milk to end up with a tasty gel.

2. Take the coconut milk gel and place it into the blender, along with chunks of cooked squash. Blend everything together to get a smooth porridge.

3. Pour the porridge into a pan and cook on medium heat. Be sure to stir frequently to avoid searing the bottom. Remove from heat when the porridge begins to bubble.

4. When serving, consider topping with nuts, berries, or any leftover gel you may have.

Banana and Blueberry Pancakes

Ingredients:

- Apple cider vinegar (1 Tbsp.)

- Baking soda (1 tsp)

- Bananas (two-thirds c., mashed)

- Cassava flour (1 c.)

- Cinnamon (2 tsp)

- Coconut milk (three-fourths c.)

- Coconut oil (2 Tbsp.)

- Coconut oil (2 Tbsp.)

- Fresh blueberries (1 c.)

- Sea salt (1 tsp)

- Tigernut flour (half c.)

Instructions:

1. Place all the ingredients except for the coconut oil into a large bowl and mix until well incorporated.

2. Use the coconut oil to grease a pan or skillet and place the pan over medium heat. Once properly heated, pour in your pancake batter, making pancakes at your preferred size and thickness.

3. When the pancakes begin to brown, and the tops have begun to bubble, flip them over, and continue to cook. The cooking process should take approximately three minutes per side.

**Cauliflower Oatmeal**

Ingredients:

- Alcohol-free vanilla extract (half tsp)

- Cauliflower (4 c., riced)

- Coconut milk (1.25 c.)

- Ground cinnamon (1 tsp)

- Himalayan pink salt

Instructions:

1. In a pan, pour in the coconut milk and mix in the vanilla extract and cinnamon. Place the pan over medium heat.

2. Allow the coconut milk to warm for a few minutes before tossing in the riced cauliflower and lower the temperature to medium-low. Be sure to stir while you wait for everything to reach a gentle simmer. Once simmering, continue cooking for five minutes.

3. When the cauliflower rice has cooked through completely, remove the pan from heat and stir in a pinch of Himalayan pink salt. Pour into bowls and serve.

**Breakfast Casserole**

Ingredients:

- Carrots (3, diced)

- Celery stalks (3, diced)

- Coconut milk (1.5 c.)

- Coconut oil (2 Tbsp.)

- Ground cinnamon (1.5 tsp)

- Mushrooms (1 lb., sliced)

- Onion (1 large, chopped)

- Onion powder (1 tsp)

- Rosemary (2 Tbsp., fresh, chopped)

- Sage (2 Tbsp., fresh, chopped)

- Sea salt (1.5 tsp)

- Spaghetti squash (1 large)

- Spinach (1 pack 10-12 oz., frozen)

- Thyme (1.5 tsp, dried)

- Zucchini (1 large, chopped)

Instructions:

1. Begin by slicing the squash in half. Remove all o the seeds. Take a baking sheet and line it with parchment paper. Roast the spaghetti squash skin side up at 400° F for 45 minutes. Once ready, shred the squash's flesh with a fork.

2. Using your preferred method, warm the frozen spinach, and drain all the extra liquid.

3. Using a tablespoon of coconut oil, sauté the celery, onion, and carrots in a pan. Make to also toss in the fresh herbs and spices.

4. In a separate pan, heat the rest of the coconut oil and sauté the mushroom and zucchini until soft. Once softened, toss in the spinach.

5. Using the bigger of the two pans, mix all of the ingredients together and add salt and pepper to your liking.

6. When the seasoning is done, take the casserole mixture and pour it into a greased baking dish or tray.

7. Heat the oven to 375° F and place the tray inside. Bake for 40 minutes or until the casserole is bubbling. Remove the casserole from the oven and allow it to cool.

8. Slice the casserole, plate, and serve.

Banana Coconut Bread

Ingredients:

- Arrowroot starch (half c.)

- Baking soda (half tsp)

- Bananas (1 c., mashed)

- Coconut butter (half c., softened)

- Coconut flour (quarter c.)

- Coconut oil (4 Tbsp., melted)

- Ground cinnamon (half tsp)

- Lemon juice (1.5 tsp)

- Maple syrup (1 Tbsp.)

- Salt (half tsp)

Instructions:

1. Get started by heating up your oven to 350° F. Take a standard 9 by 13 baking pan and crease it with the coconut oil.

2. Dump the banana, syrup, vanilla extract, juice, and butter into a stand mixer and combine until smooth. If you do not have a stand mixer, a large bowl and a hand mixer will work too.

3. Toss in the rest of the ingredients and continue to mix. Once thoroughly combined, take the batter and spread it as evenly as you can onto the greased baking pan.

4. Throw it into the oven and let it cook for about half an hour. The bread is done when you are able to stick a

toothpick or fork through it without any batter sticking
to the prongs.

5. Allow the bread to cool slightly before serving.

**Pumpkin and Pumpkin Bagels**

Ingredients:

- Arrowroot starch (three-quarters c.)

- Cassava flour (1 c.)

- Cranberries (half c., dried and unsweetened)

- Instant yeast (2.5 tsp)

- Maple syrup (1 Tbsp.)

- Pumpkin puree (quarter c.)

- Salt (1 tsp)

- Tigernut flour (1 c.)

- Warm water (1 c.)

Instructions:

1. Set your oven to 450° F and allow it to preheat. While waiting, take a baking sheet and place parchment paper over it to keep the bagels from sticking.

2. Mix the warm water with the yeast and maple syrup. Whip together the cassava, tigernut, and arrowroot flours along with salt.

3. Pour in the pumpkin puree along with three quarters of the yeast mixture you made previously. You want your dough to be tacky to the touch and able to hold its shape. If you need to adjust the amount of water added to the batter to get this consistency, do so.

4. Toss in the cranberries, stirring them around, and then knead the dough. You'll want to do this on a flat surface with a bit of flour on it.

5. Separate the dough into five pieces and begin to form bagels. Once done, get a large pot of water and get it up to boiling. You'll want enough space and water to allow the bagels to move around and not stick to one another.

6. Once boiling, place two or three bagels into the pot. Allow them to cook for roughly four minutes. The bagels will have a tendency to settle at the bottom of the pot, so keep an eye on them and dislodge them if they get stuck.

7. Pull the bagels out and place them on the pan with parchment paper. Repeat step 6 as necessary to boil all your bagels. Place the baking sheet in the oven for twenty minutes.

8. Pull the bagels out and allow them to cool before serving.

Lemon Waffles

Ingredients:

- Baking soda (half tsp)

- Ground cinnamon (quarter tsp)

- Lemon zest (1.5 tsp, finely grated)

- Olive oil (quarter c.)

- Plantains (3)

- Sea salt (half tsp)

Instructions:

1. Grab your plantains and peel them. Slice them, so they fit into a blender. Toss in the rest of the ingredients as well and blend them to create a smooth batter.

2. Prepare a waffle iron by getting it hot. Grease it with a bit of olive oil.

3. Scoop in the waffle batter using as much as you need for your specific iron.

4. Cook for roughly five minutes, or until your waffles are a nice golden color.

Sweet Potato Cookies

Ingredients:

- Coconut oil (quarter c.)

- Coconut sugar (quarter c.)

- Ground cinnamon (1 tsp)

- Ground flax seed (1 Tbsp.)

- Ground nutmeg (half tsp)

- Pumpkin seeds (quarter c.)

- Sweet potato (half c., mashed)

- Unsweetened dried coconut (1.5 c.)

Instructions:

1. Get the oven ready by setting it to 350° F. Grab a sheet pan and line it with parchment paper or lightly grease it with some coconut oil.

2. Take the ground flaxseed and mix it with three tablespoons of cold water. Chill the mixture in the fridge while the rest of the cookie batter is prepared.

3. Place the sweet potato and coconut sugar into a stand mixer bowl and beat on low. Melt the coconut oil in the microwave and slowly pour it into the potato mixture.

4. Toss in the cinnamon, nutmeg, coconut, and pumpkin seeds. Take the chilled flax seed mixture and pour it in as well. Once all the ingredients have gotten beaten together and thoroughly combined, take the dough, and shape it into balls.

5. Take the dough balls and flatten them on the sheet pan. Place the pan in the oven and allow the cookies to bake for about ten minutes or when they take on a golden-brown color.

6. Remove the cookies from heat and let them cool for five minutes, after which remove them off the tray and allow them to cool completely on a cooling or wire rack.

Tigernut Granola

Ingredients:

- Alcohol-free vanilla extract (1 tsp)

- Avocado oil (quarter c.)

- Carob powder (1 Tbsp.)

- Coconut flakes (1 c.)

- Maple syrup (quarter c.)

- Tigernuts (1 c., sliced)

Instructions:

1. Get your oven up to 275° F. While getting your oven setup, make sure that the rack you will use is in the middle rung.

2. Place all the ingredients into a bowl and thoroughly combine. Take a sheet pan and lightly grease it with avocado oil. Pour the granola mixture onto the pan, trying to spread it into a single, even layer.

3. Toss the granola into the oven and bake for half an hour. Stir every 15 minutes. This will ensure that your granola does not burn and it cooks evenly throughout.

4. Take the granola out and break apart any large chunks that may have formed. If the granola is still a bit damp after pulling it out, do not fret: the granola should finish drying out with the residual heat and as it cools off.

Apple Cinnamon Rolls

Ingredients:

- Arrowroot starch (quarter c.)

- Baking soda (half tsp)

- Coconut butter (personal preference on amount)

- Coconut flour (quarter c.)

- Coconut oil (2 Tbsp., melted)

- Granny smith apple (1 c., finely chopped)

- Ground cinnamon (2 tsp)

- Medjool dates (5, pitted)

- Sea salt (quarter tsp)

- Unsweetened applesauce (quarter c.)

- White sweet potato (2 c., peeled and diced)

Instructions:

1. Get your oven ready to bake by setting it up to 350° F.

2. Take the diced sweet potato and steam it for 15 minutes. Keep the pieces covered while they cook. The potato is done when you can break apart the pieces easily with a fork or spoon.

3. Place the sweet potato into a blender or food processor. Follow this up with the applesauce and two tablespoons of coconut oil. Blend the ingredients together until evenly mixed.

4. In a large bowl, mix the coconut flour, arrowroot starch, baking soda, salt, and cinnamon. Once everything has been evenly distributed, mix in the sweet potato.

5. Take a saucepan and scoop in the remaining coconut oil. Place it over medium-low heat and begin sauteing the apple bits. While you wait for the apple bits to soften, microwave the Medjool dates with half a cup of water for one minute.

6. Pour in the dates as well as four tablespoons of the date water, any remaining cinnamon, and salt into the pan. Crush the apple pieces and dates. Allow the juices in the pan to reduce and add the remaining date water. Simmer while constantly stirring. The liquid should reduce down to a paste. Once it does, remove the pan from heat. You now have your roll filling.

7. Take the filling and spoon it on to the dough. Roll the dough into a log or cylinder, making sure the filling is kept inside the log and evenly distributed. Have the seam on the bottom of the log.

8. Slice the dough into six even pieces. Take a baking tray and line it with parchment paper. Place the raw cinnamon rolls onto the tray and place them in the oven.

9. Bake the cinnamon rolls for 20 minutes. They should turn a nice golden-brown when done. Take your coconut butter and drizzle it over each roll before serving.

Tropical Breakfast Bowl

Ingredients:

- Dairy-free coconut yogurt (1 c.)

- Fresh mango (half a fruit, diced)

- Kiwi (1, diced and peeled)

- Maple syrup (1 tsp)

- Raspberries (2 Tbsp.)

Instructions:

1. Mix your yogurt with maple syrup. Split this in half evenly between two bowls.

2. Top each bowl with bits of kiwi and mango. Toss in some raspberries as well and enjoy.

Breakfast Vegetable Hash

Ingredients:

- Broccoli (1 head, chopped)

- Coconut oil (2 Tbsp.)

- Garlic cloves (2, crushed and minced)

- Olive oil (1 Tbsp.)

- Onion (1, diced)

- Salt (Half tsp)

- Sweet potato (1 large, diced)

Instructions:

1. Take a frying pan and grease it with coconut oil. Set it over medium heat.

2. Mince your garlic cloves and dice the onion before throwing them into your pan.

3. Take your sweet potato and remove the ends. Peel the skin and dice the potato into small, bite-sized pieces. Toss the chunks of sweet potato into the frying pan along with a bit of salt.

4. Wash your broccoli and then chop the florets into small pieces and place them into the frying pan.

5. Allow the vegetables to cook until they have softened. If you prefer your veggies browned, do so.

6. Remove from heat and drizzle olive oil over the vegetables. Plate and serve your breakfast hash.

Pumpkin and Coconut Porridge

Ingredients:

- Alcohol-free vanilla extract (1 tsp)

- Banana (1, mashed)

- Coconut flour (4 Tbsp.)

- Coconut shreds (two-thirds c.)

- Full-fat coconut milk (1 c.)

- Ground cinnamon (2 tsp)

- Ground cloves (an eighth tsp)

- Ground ginger (1 tsp)

- Pumpkin puree (1.5 c.)

- Salt

- Warm water (two-thirds c.)

Instructions:

1. In a saucepan, mix your pumpkin puree, banana, coconut flour, shredded coconut, water, coconut milk, cinnamon, cloves, ginger, and salt. Place over low heat.

2. Allow the porridge to simmer, stirring on occasion. The mixture should eventually get a consistency that is thick.

3. Scoop the porridge into a bowl and top with fruit, coconut flakes, or some maple syrup.

**Overnight Oats**

Ingredients:

- Alcohol-free vanilla extract (quarter tsp)

- Chia seeds (1 Tbsp.)

- Honey (1 Tbsp.)

- Milk (half c., your choice on variety or substitute)

- Old-fashioned whole oats (half c.)

- Plain Greek yogurt (quarter c.)

Instructions:

1. Place all the ingredients into a glass container, mixed thoroughly, and place the container in the fridge. Allow a minimum of two hours of chill time, but it will taste better if you allow it to sit overnight.

2. When serving, consider topping with berries or coconut flakes.

Apple Breakfast Casserole

Ingredients:

- Agar agar (2 Tbsp.)

- Alcohol-free vanilla extract (1 tsp)

- Apple (1, peeled and diced)

- Applesauce (half c.)

- Arrowroot starch (2 Tbsp.)

- Avocado oil (quarter c.)

- Baking soda (half tsp)

- Cream of tartar (1 tsp)

- Ground cinnamon (1.5 tsp)

- Mace (quarter tsp, ground)

- Plantain (1, mashed)

- Raisins (half c.)

- Sea salt (half tsp)

- Spaghetti squash (4 c., cooked, drained, flaked)

Instructions:

1. Combine your cinnamon, spaghetti squash, mace, plantain, applesauce, salt, vanilla extract, rains, oil, and apple bits into a large bowl. Allow the mixture to sit overnight in the fridge.

2. The following day, take the remaining ingredients and thoroughly mix them in a large bowl.

3. Prepare your oven by setting the temperature to 350° F. Grease a casserole dish with a bit of oil. Mix the dry ingredients together with the spaghetti squash mixture and spread it evenly into the casserole dish.

4. Bake for an hour. The casserole should be done when it has turned light brown, and the edges have bubbled.

<u>*Vegan Waffles*</u>

Ingredients:

- Arrowroot starch (quarter tsp)

- Avocado oil (3 Tbsp.)

- Cassava flour (1.25 c.)

- Cream of tartar (1.25 tsp)

- Ground cinnamon (1 tsp)

- Maple syrup (2 Tbsp.)

- Water (1.25 c.)

Instructions:

1. Combine all the dry ingredients in a bowl. Add the wet ingredients one at a time and slowly mix in the water. The waffle batter should be thicker than pancake mix. If you add too much water on accident, mix in a bit of cassava flour to even it out.

2. Preheat your waffle iron and grease it with a bit of oil. When hot, pour in the waffle batter.

3. Once the waffles are a nice golden color, pull them out of the iron and serve with maple syrup.

Instant Pot Quinoa

Ingredients:

- Apple cider vinegar (2 Tbsp.)

- Full-fat coconut milk (2 c.)

- Maple syrup (a third c.)

- Quinoa (2 c.)

- Water (1.5 c.)

Instructions:

1. Combine the apple cider vinegar and quinoa in a bowl. Add enough water to cover the quinoa and allow it to soak overnight.

2. Pour the quinoa into a sieve and rinse with water until it runs clear.

3. Put the quinoa into your instant pot with 1.5 cups of water.

4. Pour in two cups of the full-fat coconut milk, salt, and maple syrup.

5. Cook under high pressure for three minutes.

6. Use the natural pressure release and wait for ten minutes. Once the pressure has been fully released, scoop the quinoa into bowls and serve.

Chapter 8:
Anti-Inflammatory Lunches

You can't forget lunch. When you're halfway through your day, you need that energy boost to make it through. By following this diet and choosing these recipes, you will give yourself that powerhouse of nutrients that you will need to keep moving forward to make it to dinner. You will help yourself to prevent that afternoon crash by finding these foods and entering them into your diet.

Chow Mein

Ingredients:

- Broccoli florets (3.5 oz., chopped)

- Carrot (1, peeled and julienned)

- Coconut aminos (2 Tbsp.)

- Fresh ginger (thumb-sized chunk, peeled and minced)

- Garlic cloves (2, crushed)

- Olive oil (2 Tbsp.)

- Shirataki noodles (6 oz.)

- Sweetener of choice

Instructions:

1. Pour water into a pan and bring to a boil. Rinse the shirataki noodles and toss them into the water. After a few minutes, remove the pan from heat and set it aside.

2. Take a frying pan and pour in the olive oil. Place it over medium heat. Sauté the carrot and broccoli until softened a bit.

3. Toss in the garlic and ginger and sauté for an additional two minutes.

4. Pour in the aminos and sweetener. You want to reduce the sauce down, so increase the temperature if necessary. Be sure to stir constantly.

5. Pull the noodles out of the pan of water and add them to the stir-fried vegetables. Fry the noodles until you get your preferred doneness.

6. Remove the chow mein from heat and serve.

Braised Lamb With Fennel

Ingredients:

- Bay leaves (2)

- Chicken broth (2 c.)

- Cinnamon stick (1)

- Fennel (1 bulb, chopped)

- Garlic (1 bulb, chopped in half)

- Lamb shoulder (3 lbs., cut into eighths)

- Olive oil (2 Tbsp.)

- Onion (1, chopped)

- Orange (1, with peel, cut into wedges)

- White wine (1 c.)

- Whole peeled tomatoes (14.5 oz., can)

Instructions:

1. Dry the lamb shoulder and season with pepper and salt. Place oil in a dutch oven and sear the lamb thoroughly. Set the lamb aside on a plate.

2. Toss in garlic, onion, and fennel into the dutch oven and cook. Brown, but do not burn the ingredients, especially the garlic, or it will taste bitter. Pour in the wine and allow it to boil. This should deglaze the oven. Drop the heat and allow everything to simmer. Reduce the liquid to half of what you started with.

3. Add in the orange wedges, tomatoes, bay leaves, cinnamon, broth. Reintroduce the lamb as well. Simmer for a few minutes, then cover the dutch oven.

4. Set your oven to 325° F and bake for an hour and a half. Move the lamb onto a plate. Strain the juice in the dutch oven to remove all the solid ingredients and return the juice back to the oven. Allow it to boil until reduced and thickened. This should take about half an hour.

5. When the sauce has thickened, place the lamb back into the dutch oven to warm. Serve the lamb with plenty of sauce and enjoy.

<u>***Spaghetti With Clams***</u>

Ingredients:

- Clams (6.5 lbs.)

- Olive oil (6 Tbsp.)

- White wine (0.5 c.)

- Garlic clove (3, sliced)

- Chiles (3, small and crumbled)

- Spaghetti (1 lb.)

- Fresh Parsley (3 Tbsp., chopped)

- Salt and pepper

Instructions:

1. Take the clams and soak them in clean water. Use a brush to clean them and remove any dirt or sand stuck on the shells.

2. Use two tablespoons of olive oil to grease a large pot. Pour in half of your wine, one of the garlic cloves, and one of the chilies. Cook half of the clams, shaking them on occasion until they open. Pull out the clams as they open and toss in fresh clams. If a clam refuses to open, throw it away.

3. Prepare the spaghetti pasta using the packaging instructions and cook it until al dente. Save a cup of the pasta water.

4. Place a pot over medium heat and throw in the remaining chile and garlic. Sauté for two minutes and then dump the clams and their juice in. Pour in the

pasta and toss. Use pasta water to deglaze your pot as necessary.

5. Serve and season with pepper and salt. Garnish with parsley.

Curried Cauliflower Rice

Ingredients:

- Cauliflower (1 head)

- Cinnamon powder (half tsp)

- Coconut oil (2 Tbsp.)

- Fresh parsley (quarter c., chopped)

- Garlic powder (1 tsp)

- Ginger (quarter tsp)

- Lemon juice (2 tsp)

- Olives (half c.)

- Onion powder (1 tsp)

- Sea salt

- Turmeric powder (1.5 tsp)

Instructions:

1. Take your cauliflower to a grater or process it in a blender to get rice-like bits.

2. Set a pan over high heat and warm the coconut oil. Once melted and the pan is coated well, toss in the cauliflower rice. Sauté for five minutes, making sure to stir often.

3. Toss in the spices and coat your rice thoroughly. Continue to sauté for another three minutes.

4. Pour in the olives and allow them to cook for a minute.

5. Remove the pan off the burner and serve the cauliflower rice. Use freshly chopped parsley to garnish.

Ratatouille

Ingredients:

- Carrots (3, peeled and chopped)

- Dried oregano (1 Tbsp.)

- Fresh rosemary (1 Tbsp., minced)

- Garlic cloves (4, minced)

- Golden beets (2, peeled and chopped)

- Olive oil (3 Tbsp.)

- Salt

- Summer squash (1, chopped)

- Yellow onion (1, peeled and chopped)

Instructions:

1. Take a large saucepan and place it over medium-low heat. Pour in the olive oil and get it hot. Toss in the garlic, beets, and carrots and allow them to sauté for 20 minutes, stirring occasionally.

2. Toss in the onion, oregano, rosemary, squash, and zucchini. Continue cooking for another 20 minutes. Stir more frequently during this step to avoid burning or charring.

3. Adjust the seasoning as necessary and serve.

___Mulligatawny___

Ingredients:

- Apples (2, diced)

- Avocado oil (1 Tbsp.)

- Cabbage (half of one head, shredded)

- Cauliflower (half of one head, chopped)

- Cilantro (1 Tbsp.)

- Cinnamon (1 tsp)

- Cloves (quarter tsp)

- Coconut milk (1 c.)

- Fenugreek (half tsp)

- Garlic cloves (4, minced)

- Ginger (2 tsp)

- Lime (1, juiced)

- Mace (quarter tsp)

- Onion (1, diced)

- Sweet potato (1, diced)

- Turmeric (2 Tbsp.)

- Veggie broth (1 quart)

Instructions:

1. Saute the onion, ginger, garlic, turmeric, cinnamon, cilantro, mace, cloves, and fenugreek for a minute.

2. Toss in the rest of the veggies and cook for ten minutes.

3. Pour in the vegetable broth and season with pepper and salt. Allow the broth to boil, then reduce the heat and simmer. Simmer as long as it takes for the vegetables to get tender.

4. Pour in the milk as well as lime juice. Adjust the seasoning and serve.

Coconut Curry

Ingredients:

- Avocado oil (2 Tbsp.)

- Cilantro (to taste—garnish)

- Coconut milk (1 can)

- Garlic (4 cloves, minced)

- Ginger (5 g, minced or grated)

- Onion (1, peeled and chopped roughly)

- Salt

- Turmeric powder (1 Tbsp.)

- White mushrooms (20, roughly chopped)

- Zucchini (2, chunked)

Instructions:

1. Get a large frying pan and heat half of your oil over medium heat. Sauté the zucchini and mushrooms until the zucchini chunks begin to caramelize and turn a nice golden color. Remove them from the pan and set them aside.

2. Pour the remaining oil into the frying pan and sauté the onions until soft, then stir in the garlic and ginger. Continue cooking until the onions caramelize.

3. Shake in the turmeric powder and also mix in the vegetables.

4. Pour in the coconut milk and cook until thoroughly warmed. Reduce the heat to allow the curry to simmer and get thicker.

5. Remove the curry from heat and serve over rice or riced cauliflower.

Spinach Tacos

Ingredients:

- Cauliflower (2 c.)

- Coconut flour (1 Tbsp.)

- Coconut milk (1 Tbsp.)

- Coconut oil (1 Tbsp.)

- Parsnip (1 c.)

- Plantain flour (3 Tbsp.)

- Salt

- Spinach (2 c.)

Instructions:

1. Take a large frying pan and grease it with a bit of oil. Toss your veggies in and cook them until softened.

2. Take the softened parsnip and blend it in a food processor until smooth. Pour in the plantain flour and melted coconut oil. Add salt as necessary. Mix the ingredients together.

3. Move the pseudo-dough and separate it out into balls. You will smash these into tortillas. Place your tortillas on a baking sheet lined with parchment paper and bake at 350° F. They should be ready in ten minutes, but remove them early if they get crispy.

4. While waiting for the tortillas, blend the cauliflower and coconut milk with some salt, pulsing until smooth.

5. Pull the tortillas out of the oven and begin serving by spreading cauliflower sauce inside each tortilla and filling them up with spinach.

94

Baked Cod

Ingredients:

- Basil (half tsp., dried)

- Bay leaf (1)

- Capers (1 small jar)

- Cod fillets (2 pounds)

- Diced tomatoes (16-oz. can, saving the juice)

- Dry white wine (1 c.)

- Fennel seeds (1 tsp., crushed)

- Garlic (1 clove, minced)

- Lemon juice (quarter c., fresh)

- Olive oil (2 tsp)

- Onion (1, sliced)

- Orange juice (quarter c., fresh)

- Orange peel (1 Tbsp.)

- Oregano (half tsp., dried)

- Salt and pepper

Instructions:

1. Using a cast-iron skillet, warm your oil and sauté the onion for five minutes. Once done, toss in all the ingredients save for the cod fillets. Simmer for half an hour.

2. Set your oven to 375° F and allow it to preheat while finishing the sauce.

3. Place the fillets into the cast iron and spoon the sauce over the fish. Throw the skillet into the oven and bake for 15 minutes. Once the fish flakes easily, remove it from the oven and serve.

Lemon Herb Chicken and Potatoes

Ingredients:

- Baby potatoes (8, halved)

- Basil (3 tsp, dried)

- Bell pepper (1, seeds removed and wedged)

- Chicken thighs (4, skin and bone on)

- Garlic (4 large cloves, crushed)

- Kalamata olives (4 Tbsp., pitted)

- Lemon juice (from 1 lemon)

- Lemons for garnish

- Olive oil (3 Tbsp.)

- Oregano (2 tsp, dried)

- Parsley (2 tsp, dried)

- Red onion (wedged)

- Red wine vinegar (1 Tbsp.)

- Salt (2 tsp)

- Zucchini (1 large, sliced)

Instructions:

1. Mix the lemon juice, vinegar, seasonings, garlic, and two tablespoons of olive oil in a dish. Take half of the lemon juice mixture and marinate the chicken in it for at least fifteen minutes, though overnight is preferred.

2. Set the oven to 430° F. While the oven is preheating, sear the chicken in a cast-iron skillet (or an oven-safe frying pan) with the rest of the olive oil. Drain the extra fat and oil, leaving behind only about a tablespoon of fat.

3. Place the veggies around the chicken thighs and pour the rest of the marinade on top. Cover the skillet and place it in the oven. Bake for half an hour or until the vegetables have softened and the chicken is cooked through. Remove the lid and boil for five minutes or until the chicken thighs have their skin turn golden brown and have crisped. Remove from heat and serve.

Sheet-Pan Shrimp

Ingredients:

For the shrimp

- Feta cheese (half c.)

- Fingerling potatoes (2 c., halved)

- Green beans (6 oz., trimmed)

- Olive oil (3 Tbsp.)

- Pepper (1 tsp)

- Red onion (1 medium, sliced)

- Red pepper (1 medium, sliced)

- Salt (1 tsp)

- Shrimp (1 lb., deveined and peeled)

For the Marinade

- Garlic (1 Tbsp., minced)

- Oregano (half tsp)

- Greek yogurt (1 c.)

- Lemon juice (2 Tbsp.)

- Paprika (half tsp)

- Parsley (2 Tbsp., chopped)

Instructions:

1. Mix the marinade ingredients together in a bowl and set it off to the side.

2. Marinade the shrimp in a bowl with half a cup of the lemon juice mixture. Allow it to sit for at least half an hour.

3. Get a baking sheet and line it with parchment paper or aluminum foil. Set your oven to 400° F. Prepare the vegetables while the oven is preheating and place them onto the sheet pan. Pour olive oil over them and give them a quick dusting of salt and pepper.

4. Place the sheet pan into the oven and bake for twenty minutes and then pull the veggies out. Remove the green beans, so they don't burn with the next step.

5. Make a single layer of shrimp on the baking sheet and place it back into the oven. Bake for ten minutes or until the shrimp is done. Serve in bowls and top with feta cheese and a small scoop of the marinade.

Chicken and Chickpea Soup

Ingredients:

- Artichoke hearts (14 oz. can drain and chopped)

- Bay leaf (1)

- Cayenne (quarter tsp)

- Chicken thighs (2 lbs., skins removed)

- Cumin (4 tsp)

- Diced tomatoes (1 15-oz. can)

- Dried chickpeas (1.5 c., soaked overnight)

- Garlic cloves (4, chopped)

- Olives (quarter c., halved)

- Paprika (4 tsp)

- Pepper (quarter tsp)

- Salt (half tsp)

- Tomato paste (2 Tbsp.)

- Water (4 c.)

- Yellow onion (chopped)

- Parsley or cilantro (for garnish)

Instructions:

1. Start by draining the chickpeas you soaked and throw them into a slow cooker. Add in the onions, water, garlic, tomatoes (and their juice), the seasonings, and

tomato paste. Stir everything together and insert the chicken thighs.

2. Set the slow cooker to low and cook for eight hours. If you are in a rush, cook or our hours on the high setting.

3. Pull out the chicken thighs and allow them to cool before deboning and chopping the meat. While cooling the chicken, pull out the bay leaf and add the olives and artichoke. When you are done chopping up the chicken, pour the bits back into the soup. Stir everything together and serve with a cilantro or parsley garnish.

Mediterranean Salad With Grilled Chicken

Ingredients:

- Artichoke hearts (one-third c., chopped)
- Balsamic vinegar (2 Tbsp.)
- Basil (1 tsp, dried)
- Chicken breasts (3, cut into bite-sized chunks)
- Cucumber (three-quarters c., diced)
- Feta cheese (quarter c.)
- Garlic (1 clove, minced)
- Greek yogurt (2 Tbsp.)
- Green onions (quarter c., chopped)
- Kalamata olives (3 Tbsp., sliced)
- Kosher salt (half tsp)
- Lemon juice (3 Tbsp + 1 tsp.)
- Olive oil (3 Tbsp. + 2 Tbsp.)
- Onion powder (half tsp)
- Parsley (half tsp)
- Pesto (4 tsp)
- Pinch of crushed red pepper
- Roasted red bell pepper (6 Tbsp., sliced)
- Romaine (4 c., chopped)

- Shiitake mushrooms

- Spinach (4 c., chopped)

- Tomato (three-quarters c., diced)

- White wine vinegar (4 tsp)

Instructions:

1. Mix a teaspoon of lemon juice, pesto, and wine vinegar in a mason jar or something with a lid. Shake it up to combine the ingredients. Scoop in the yogurt and two tablespoons of olive oil, again, shaking to combine. Set the vinaigrette aside.

2. Marinate your chicken breasts in three tablespoons of lemon juice, the rest of the olive oil, the seasonings, and balsamic vinegar. Allow the chicken to marinate at least half an hour, though longer is better. Soak wooden skewers in water while the chicken marinates to better protect them from charring.

3. Take the skewers and alternate poking chicken and mushroom to make kebabs. Grill the kebabs for ten minutes or until the chicken is fully cooked.

4. Create the salad by making a layer of romaine and spinach on each plate and top it with tomato, cucumber, artichoke, olives, cheese, and red pepper slices.

5. Drizzle the vinaigrette over the salad and top it with a kebab.

Slow-Cooked Brisket

Ingredients:

- Beef broth (half c.)

- Brisket (3 lbs.)

- Cold water (quarter c.)

- Fennel bulbs (2, cored, trimmed, and cut into wedges)

- Flour

- Italian seasoning (3 tsp)

- Italian seasoning diced tomatoes (one 14.5 oz. can)

- Lemon peel (1 tsp., finely shredded)

- Olives (half c.)

- Parsley for garnish

- Pepper

- Salt

Instructions:

1. Trim the excess fat and silver-skin from the beef and rub with a teaspoon of Italian seasoning. Place it into the slow cooker, topping with the fennel.

2. Pour in the tomatoes, lemon zest, broth, salt, pepper, olives, and the remaining Italian seasoning.

3. Set the slow cooker to low and cook for ten hours. If you are in a rush, set the slow cooker to high and cook for only five hours.

4. Remove the brisket from the slow cooker and place it and the veggies on a serving dish.

5. Skim the fat off the top of the juices still in the slow cooker. Take two cups of the juice and place it in a saucepan. Cook over medium heat. Mix the flour with some cold water, then pour the mixture into the meat juice. Whisk together and cook until you get a thick gravy.

6. When serving, garnish with parsley and serve with a healthy portion of gravy.

Herbed Lamb and Vegetables

Ingredients:

- Bell pepper (2, any color, seeds removed and cut into bite-sized chunks)

- Lamb cutlets (8 leans)

- Mint (2 Tbsp., fresh, chopped)

- Olive oil (1 Tbsp.)

- Red onion (1, wedged)

- Sweet potato (1 large, peeled, and chunked)

- Thyme (1 Tbsp., fresh, chopped)

- Zucchini (2, chunked)

Instructions:

1. Get your oven ready for baking by setting it to 400° F. Take a baking sheet and grease it with olive oil. Arrange the vegetables onto the baking sheet into a single layer. Crack some black pepper over them if you wish. Place the baking sheet into the oven and bake the vegetables for about half an hour.

2. While the vegetables are baking, trim the fat from the lamb cutlets. Take the herbs and mix them together with some black pepper. Rub the lamb thoroughly with the seasoning.

3. Pull the vegetables out of the oven and flip them over. Push them over to one side of the baking sheet and place the lamb onto the other side. Bake the lamb for

ten minutes and flip it. Bake for another ten minutes before pulling everything out of the oven and serving.

<u>***Harissa Pasta***</u>

Ingredients:

- Harissa paste (4 Tbsp.)

- Pasta (4 cups)

- Pine nuts (4 Tbsp.)

- Red bell pepper (2)

- Red onion (2)

Instructions:

1. Take an oven-safe baking dish or sheet pan and grease it with a bit of olive oil. Roast the peppers and onions for twenty minutes in the oven at 400° F.

2. While the veggies are roasting, prepare the pasta according to the packaging instructions.

3. While you are cooking your pasta, toast the pine nuts in a frying pan, stopping once browned.

4. Drain the pasta reserving a bit of the water. Dice the roasted vegetables and toss them into the pasta along with the Harissa paste. When serving, top with the toasted pine nuts.

Rosemary Salmon With Walnut Crust

Ingredients:

- Cooking spray

- Dijon mustard (2 tsp)

- Garlic (1 clove, minced)

- Honey (half tsp)

- Kosher salt (half tsp)

- Lemon juice (1 tsp)

- Lemon zest (quarter tsp.)

- Olive oil (1 tsp)

- Panko (3 Tbsp.)

- Parsley and lemon to garnish

- Red pepper (quarter tsp)

- Rosemary (1 tsp, chopped)

- Salmon (1 pound, skin removed)

- Walnuts (3 Tbsp., finely chopped)

Instructions:

1. Combine your mustard, lemon juice and zest, honey, red pepper, salt, and rosemary. In another bowl, mix the panko with the walnuts and olive oil.

2. Take the mustard mixture and spread it on the salmon fillet. Top the fillet with the walnut-panko mixture.

Spray down the salmon with a bit of cooking spray to really crisp up the panko.

3. Bake in the oven at 425° F. The fish is done cooking when the skin can flake easily. When serving, garnish with parsley and a few thin slices of lemon.

Easy Mediterranean Pasta Salad

Ingredients:

- Artichoke hearts (6 oz. jar, drained)

- Balsamic vinegar (1 Tbsp.)

- Kalamata olives (6-oz. jar, drained and chopped)

- Olive oil (1 Tbsp.)

- Pasta (4 oz., wheat)

- Salt

- Sun-dried tomatoes in oil (three-quarters oz. jarred, drained)

Instructions:

1. Cook your pasta to al dente using the instructions on the packaging. Toss olives, artichoke, and tomatoes together.

2. Drain the pasta and add it to a bowl with the olive mixture. Top with olive oil and vinegar before serving.

Garlic Baked Salmon With Coriander

Ingredients:

- Fresh coriander (stems trimmed)

- Garlic (4 cloves, chopped)

- Lime (half a fruit, cut into rounds)

- Lime juice (1 lime's worth)

- Olive oil (half c.)

- Salmon fillet (2 pounds, skin removed)

- Salt

- Tomato (cut into rounds)

Instructions:

1. Set your oven to 425° F. While the oven preheats, pull your salmon out and let it come up to room temperature.

2. Using a food processor or blender, blend the garlic, lime juice, coriander, salt, and olive oil.

3. Grease a baking sheet with a bit of olive oil and place the salmon fillet on it. Dust it with salt and pepper. Spread the garlic sauce over the salmon, making sure to coat it entirely. Top with tomato and lime slices.

4. Bake for ten minutes or until the salmon flakes easily. Pull the salmon out of the oven and allow it to rest before serving.

Moroccan Lentil Soup

Ingredients:

- Carrots (2 c., chopped)

- Cauliflower (3 c.)

- Cinnamon (quarter tsp)

- Cumin (1 tsp)

- Diced tomato (28 oz. from a can)

- Fresh cilantro (half c.)

- Fresh spinach (4 c.)

- Garlic (4 cloves, minced)

- Ground coriander (1 tsp)

- Lemon juice (2 Tbsp.)

- Lentils (1.75 c.)

- Olive oil (2 tsp)

- Onion (2 c., chopped)

- Pepper

- Tomato paste (2 Tbsp.)

- Turmeric (1 tsp)

- Vegetable broth (6 c.)

- Water (2 c.)

Instructions:

1. Save for the spinach, lemon juice, and cilantro, mix all the ingredients together in a slow cooker. Cook on low for ten hours or until the lentils have softened. If you are in a hurry, cook for five hours on the high setting.

2. When there's only half an hour left on the timer, toss in the spinach.

3. When serving, garnish with cilantro and a bit of lemon juice.

Chapter 9:
Anti-Inflammatory Dinners

Dinner is perhaps the most important meal socially in our current culture. When we get home for dinner, we all sit around the table to enjoy our time together, catching up with our family and socializing. It is that act of reconnecting from a busy day so that we can enjoy ourselves and relax with our loved ones. It can be all too easy to be tempted into just ordering something easy to eat so that you don't have to cook, but that's why you have this chapter with all of these healthy, anti-inflammatory recipes that will help you to ensure that at the end of the day, you have options that will be easy to throw together. Some of these can be made ahead, while others can be tossed into the slow cooker first thing in the morning to be ready when you need them.

Mediterranean Mahi Mahi

Ingredients:

- Basil (6 leaves, freshly chopped)

- Capers (4 Tbsp.)

- Garlic (2 cloves, chopped)

- Italian seasoning (a dash)

- Kalamata olives (25, chopped)

- Lemon juice (1 tsp)

- Mahi mahi (1 lb.)

- Olive oil (2 Tbsp.)

- Onion (half a bulb, chopped)

- Parmesan cheese (3 Tbsp.)

- Diced tomatoes (15 oz. can)

- White wine (quarter c.)

Instructions:

1. Take a frying pan and place your olive oil in. Warm over medium heat. Cook the diced onion until transparent. Mix in the Italian seasoning and garlic.

2. Pour in the can of tomatoes, olives, wine, and half of the basil. Reduce the heat and sprinkle in the parmesan cheese. Remove the pan from heat once the mixture bubbles.

3. Grease a baking sheet with a bit of oil and arrange the mahi mahi on it. Top with the sauce you just finished making. Bake for twenty minutes at 425° F or until the fish flakes easily.

Slow-Cooked Mediterranean Chicken

Ingredients:

- Bay leaf (1)

- Capers (1 Tbsp.)

- Chicken broth (half c.)

- Chicken thighs (2 pounds, boneless and skinless)

- Garlic (3 cloves, minced)

- Kalamata olives (1 c.)

- Olive oil (1 Tbsp.)

- Oregano (1 tsp)

- Roasted red pepper (1 c.)

- Rosemary (1 tsp, dried)

- Salt and pepper

- Sweet onion (1, thinly sliced)

- Thyme (1 tsp, dried)

Instructions:

1. In a frying pan over medium-high heat, sauté the chicken with the olive oil. Make sure to brown both sides. Set the chicken aside and then sauté the garlic and onions until transparent.

2. Throw all the ingredients into the slow cooker and set it to low. Cook for four hours. Check the seasoning and adjust accordingly before serving.

Greek Stuffed Mushrooms

Ingredients:

- Cherry tomatoes (1 c., quartered)

- Feta cheese (two-thirds c.)

- Garlic cloves (2, minced)

- Ground pepper (1 tsp)

- Kalamata olives (4 Tbsp.)

- Olive oil (6 Tbsp.)

- Oregano (2 Tbsp., fresh and roughly chopped)

- Portobello mushrooms (8, cleaned with stems and gills taken out)

- Salt (half tsp)

- Spinach (2 c., chopped)

Instructions:

1. Get your oven preheated up to 400° F.

2. Mix the salt, garlic, four tablespoons of olive oil, and half a teaspoon of pepper and rub this all over the mushrooms.

3. Lightly grease a baking sheet and arrange the mushrooms on it. Place in the oven and bake for ten to twelve minutes.

4. Combine the rest of the ingredients. Remove the mushrooms from the oven and stuff them with the filling. Stick the baking sheet back into the oven and cook for a final ten minutes.

Garlic-Roasted Salmon With Brussels Sprouts

Ingredients:

- Brussels sprouts (6 c., trimmed and halved)

- Chardonnay (three-quarters c.)

- Garlic cloves (14 large)

- Olive oil (quarter c.)

- Oregano (2 Tbsp., fresh)

- Pepper (three-quarters tsp)

- Salmon fillet (2 lbs., skin-off—cut in 6 pieces)

- Salt (1 tsp)

- Lemon wedges to serve

Instructions:

1. Begin by mincing two garlic cloves and combining them with the olive oil. Mix this together with a tablespoon of oregano, a third of the pepper, and half the salt. Dice the remaining garlic cloves and set them aside.

2. Use three tablespoons of the garlic oil pour it into a roasting pan. Toss in the garlic you saved and the brussels sprouts and roast them for fifteen minutes at 450° F in your oven.

3. Mix in the chardonnay to the rest of the garlic oil. Pull the baking sheet out of the oven and stir the vegetables. Place the salmon on top of the veggies and pour the wine-oil over it. Dust the salmon with the remaining salt, pepper, and oregano.

4. Place the baking sheet back into the oven and cook for an additional ten minutes.

Vegetarian Zucchini Lasagna Rolls

Ingredients:

- Basil (2 Tbsp., fresh)

- Egg (1, lightly beaten)

- Frozen spinach (10-ounce package, thawed and dried)

- Garlic (1 clove)

- Marinara sauce (three-quarters c.)

- Olive oil (2 tsp)

- Parmesan cheese (3 Tbsp.)

- Pepper

- Ricotta (one and a third c.)

- Salt

- Shredded mozzarella cheese (8 Tbsp.)

- Zucchini (2, trimmed)

Instructions:

1. Grease two baking sheets with oil or cooking spray. Preheat the oven to 425° F.

2. Cut the zucchini into strips longways. Aim for an eighth of an inch thickness.

3. Coat the zucchini strips with salt, pepper, and olive oil. Arrange a single layer on one sheet pan. Bake it in the oven for ten minutes or until soft.

4. Blend two tablespoons of mozzarella and a tablespoon of parmesan cheeses. In a bowl, meld the egg, spinach, garlic, ricotta, and the remaining cheese. Throw in a dash of salt and pepper.

5. In a casserole dish, spread a quarter cup of marinara sauce spread on the bottom.

6. Roll the softened zucchini strips with a tablespoon of ricotta mix at the center. Place the zucchini rolls with the seam down on the marinara. Continue this step until you run out of space or out of zucchini.

7. Top the rolls with the rest of the marinara sauce and a layer of the cheese blend.

8. Bake in the oven for twenty minutes. Let it rest for five minutes after removing from heat and top with fresh basil.

Mediterranean Chicken and Couscous Wraps

Ingredients:

- Chicken tenders (1 pound)
- Couscous (one-third c.)
- Cucumber (1, chopped)
- Garlic cloves (2 tsp, minced)
- Lemon juice (one-quarter c.)
- Mint (half c., fresh chopped)
- Olive oil (3 Tbsp.)
- Parsley (1 c., fresh and chopped)
- Pepper
- Salt
- Spinach wraps (4, 10-inch)
- Tomato (1, chopped)
- Water (half c)

Instructions:

1. Begin by cooking the couscous according to the directions on the packaging.

2. Combine the lemon juice, garlic, oil, salt, pepper, parsley, and mint.

3. Coat the chicken tenders with a tablespoon of the lemon juice mixture and sprinkle with a bit more salt.

Cook on a frying pan over medium heat until cook through.

4. Allow the chicken to cool and cube it.

5. Pour the parsley mixture into the couscous with the tomato and cucumber pieces.

6. When serving, place three-quarters of a cup of the couscous mix into a spinach wrap, finishing with chicken bits before rolling and plating.

Cheesy Artichoke and Spinach Stuffed Squash

Ingredients:

- Artichoke Hearts (10 oz., frozen-thawed and chopped up)

- Basil (for garnish)

- Black pepper

- Cream cheese (4 oz., softened)

- Crushed red pepper (for garnish)

- Parmesan cheese (0.5 c.)

- Salt

- Spaghetti squash (1, cut in half and cleaned out of seeds)

- Spinach (5 oz.)

- Water (3 Tbsp.)

Instructions:

1. Soften your squash by microwaving it sliced side down along with two tablespoons of water for ten to fifteen minutes.

2. Mix the spinach and remaining water into a frying pan until the spinach wilts. Drain and set aside.

3. Set your oven to broil with a rack set on the top rung. Combine the artichoke, salt, pepper, cheeses. Spread on the flesh of the squash halves.

4. Broil the squash shell side down for three minutes and garnish with basil and crushed red pepper.

<u>*Bean and Spinach Soup*</u>

Ingredients:

- Basil (1 tsp., dried)

- Black pepper

- Garlic (2 cloves, minced)

- Great Northern or White beans (one 15-oz. can)

- Onion (half c., chopped)

- Salt

- Spinach (8 c., chopped)

- Tomato puree (one 15-oz. can)

- Vegetable broth (three 14-oz. cans)

- White rice (half c)

Instructions:

1. Save for the spinach, throw all the ingredients into a slow cooker. Set the device to low and cook for seven hours. If you are in a rush, cook for two and a half hours on the high setting.

2. Toss in the spinach and allow it to wilt before serving.

Vegan Mediterranean Pasta

Ingredients:

- Artichokes (half c.)

- Basil leaves (quarter c., torn)

- Black pepper

- Garlic cloves (2-3 to taste, minced)

- Grape tomatoes (2 c., halved)

- Kalamata olives (10, pitted)

- Olive oil (1 Tbsp.)

- Pasta (8 oz.)

- Red pepper (quarter tsp.)

- Salt

- Spinach (4 c.)

- Tomato paste (4 Tbsp.)

- Vegetable broth (1 c.)

Instructions:

1. Cook the pasta to al dente according to the package's instructions. Reserve a cup of the pasta water for use later. Set the pasta aside.

2. Set a frying pan over medium heat with olive oil. Sauté the garlic and red pepper. Pour in the tomato paste and cook for about a minute. Toss in the grape tomatoes, artichokes, olives, broth, and seasonings. Cook until the grape tomatoes start to melt down.

3. Toss in the pasta and cook for two minutes. If the tomato sauce reduces too much, pour in some pasta water that you saved from earlier.

4. Mix in the spinach and basil. Remove from heat when they wilt.

**Shrimp Stir Fry**

Ingredients:

- Bird's eye chili (2)

- Buckwheat noodles (5 oz.)

- Celery (two-thirds c., chopped)

- Chicken stock (1 c.)

- Garlic (2 cloves)

- Ginger (2 tsp. minced)

- Green beans (1 c., chopped)

- Kale (1.5 c., chopped)

- Olive oil (4 Tbsp.)

- Red onion (one-third c., diced)

- Shelled shrimp (2 c.)

- Soy sauce (4 Tbsp.)

Instructions:

1. Set a frying pan over medium heat. Use half of your oil and soy sauce for cooking the shrimp.

2. Set the shrimp and juices aside. Wipe down the pan for use in a minute.

3. Cook the buckwheat noodles to al dente according to the instructions on the packaging. Set them aside.

4. Pour the remaining oil into the pan and toss in all the veggies. Cook over medium-high heat for a few minutes. Add the chicken stock at this point.

5. Get the stock up to boiling before lowering the temperature to get it to simmer. Throw in the noodles and shrimp. Increase the temperature for a brief period just to get everything boiling again.

6. Remove from heat and serve.

Spiced Chicken Cauliflower Couscous

Ingredients:

- Birds eye chili (2, diced)

- Capers (2 Tbsp.)

- Carrots (half c., diced)

- Cauliflower (3 c., riced)

- Chicken breast (2)

- Garlic (2 cloves, minced)

- Ginger (2 tsp, minced)

- Olive oil (4 Tbsp.)

- Lemon juice (from a whole lemon)

- Parsley (20 sprigs, chopped)

- Red onions (half c., diced)

- Sun-dried tomatoes (half c.)

- Turmeric powder (4 tsp)

Instructions:

1. Chop the florets of the cauliflower into chunks and throw them into a food processor. Pulse to get rice bits.

2. In a frying pan, heat up olive oil over medium-high heat. When ready, sauté the onions, ginger, garlic, and chili.

3. Shake in the turmeric and add in the cauliflower rice and carrot chunks. Cook until the veggies have softened.

4. Remove from heat and set the food aside in a bowl. Mix in the sun-dried tomatoes and parsley.

5. Using the same frying pan, pour in the remaining oil and cook the chicken over medium heat. Once the chicken is cooked through, pour in the lemon juice, water, and capers. After two minutes of cooking, mix in the cauliflower rice and sauce. Remove from heat and serve. Garnish with fresh cilantro.

Chicken and Kale Curry

Ingredients:

- Cardamoms (2, whole)

- Cayenne powder (1 tsp)

- Chicken thighs (4, boneless, skinless, cubed)

- Cinnamon (1 stick)

- Cloves (2, whole)

- Coconut milk (half c., canned)

- Coriander powder (4 tsp)

- Fennel seed (quarter tsp)

- Garlic cloves (4, crushed and minced)

- Ginger (1 tsp)

- Kale (4 leaves, chopped and de-stemmed)

- Olive oil (3 Tbsp.)

- Red onion (2 c., chopped)

- Salt

- Tomato (1 c., chopped)

- Turmeric (half tsp)

- Water (1 c.)

Instructions:

1. Use an instant pot for this recipe and set it to the sauté setting. Toss in the whole spices and olive oil. After a

few minutes of this, add the onion, garlic, and ginger into the mix.

2. When the onions are transparent, mix in the powdered spices, coriander, and tomato. Sauté until the tomatoes are soft. Make sure to stir regularly to avoid burning anything.

3. Turn the instant pot off and toss in the chicken, coconut milk, salt, kale, and water. Set the cooking time to five minutes manually and seal the pot.

4. When time is up, change the setting to warm and allow the curry to cook for four more minutes. Open the release valve and then quick release the instant pot's pressure.

5. Give the curry a taste and add more seasonings, as necessary. Serve over rice or noodles.

Turmeric Baked Salmon

Serves: 2

Time: 35 minutes

Ingredients:

- Birds eye chili (1, minced)

- Canned green lentils (2/3 c.)

- Celery (3 cups, chopped)

- Chicken stock (1 c.)

- Curry powder (2 tsp)

- Garlic (2 cloves, minced)

- Lemon juice (half lemon)

- Olive oil (2 tsp)

- Parsley (2 Tbsp. chopped)

- Red onion (c., diced)

- Salmon (8 oz., skinned)

- Tomatoes (3, diced)

- Turmeric powder (2 tsp)

Instructions:

1. Ensure your oven is at 400F.

2. Over medium-low heat, pour olive oil into a frying pan until oil is shimmery within the pan. Toss in onion, garlic, celery, ginger, and chilis to soften them. Toss in curry powder and wait for 3 minutes.

3. Include your tomatoes, stock, and lentils. Simmer for 10 minutes until celery is to your liking.

4. Mix in turmeric, lemon, and oil into a small jar. Then, cover the salmon with it, and put the salmon on a baking tray. Cook until flaky (10 minutes). Top with parsley and serve together.

Miso Tofu Stir Fry

Serves: 4

Time: 40 minutes

Ingredients:

- Birds eye chili (2)
- Brown miso paste (2 Tbsp.)
- Buckwheat noodles (half c.)
- Celery (1 stalk, finely chopped)
- Garlic (2 cloves, minced)
- Kale (1.25 c., ribs removed)
- Olive oil (4 tsp)
- Red onion (1, sliced thinly)
- Sesame seeds (4 tsp)
- Soy sauce (2 tsp)
- Tofu (1 package)
- Turmeric powder (2 tsp)
- Water (1 c.)
- White wine (2 Tbsp.)
- Zucchini (1, sliced thinly)

Instructions:

1. Prep your baking sheet while the oven warms to 400F.

2. Mix miso paste and wine together and set aside. Then, set the mixture to the side. Cut up tofu into triangles and marinate in the mixture.

3. Steam your kale, pulling off the heat when wilting.

4. Slice veggies and set aside.

5. Put the tofu on a baking sheet, then top with sesame seeds.

6. Bake the tofu for 20 minutes, stopping if you notice the surface already caramelized.

7. Prepare buckwheat noodles according to directions.

8. When you have five minutes until tofu is done, sauté veggies in olive oil. Serve everything together.

Sweet Potato Cauliflower Soup

Serves: 12

Time: 1 hour

Ingredients:

- Cauliflower (2 heads, chopped)

- Olive oil

- Sweet potatoes (6, cubed)

- Sweet onion (2, diced)

- Garlic cloves (4)

- Water (14 c.)

- Salt (1.5 tsp)

Instructions:

1. Set your oven to 400F. Then, spread cauliflower, coating in olive oil, onto a baking sheet. Allow it to bake for 20 minutes.

2. While the cauliflower cools, prepare a pot with onion, garlic, and potatoes boiling in water. Toss in the salt.

3. Reduce heat and simmer until potatoes are soft. Toss in cauliflower. Then, divide the soup into two batches.

4. Blend half of the soup and then mix it into the other. Add salt to taste. Enjoy!

**Pajeon**

Serves: 4

Time: 1 hour

Ingredients:

- Cassava flour (1.5 c.)

- Sea salt (1 tsp)

- Baking Soda (1 tsp)

- Olive oil (2 Tbsp.)

- Cold water (2.5 c.)

- Scallions (1 bunch, sliced)

- Carrot (1, julienned)

- Zucchini (1, julienned)

- Garlic cloves (3, chopped)

- Apple cider vinegar (1 Tbsp.)

- Coconut oil

Instructions:

1. Warm a skillet to medium heat. Mix all ingredients into a dough. Add water if necessary to make a batter that will spoon easily without being runny.

2. Put 1 c. batter onto greased skillet. Cook until brown, then flip when both sides are brown, top with scallions.

Mushroom Ravioli

Serves:

Time:

Ingredients:

Dough:

- *Tigernut flour (1 c.)*
- *Cassava flour (1 c.)*
- *Tapioca flour (.5 c.)*
- *Sea salt (1.5 c.)*
- *EVOO (2 Tbsp.)*
- *Nutritional yeast(2Tbsp.)*
- *Ground Turmeric (.5 tsp)*
- *Hot water (.75 c.)*
- *Tapioca flour*

Filling:

- Olive oil (2 Tbsp.)
- Mushrooms (3 cups)
- Onion (1)
- Garlic (4 cloves)
- Apple cider vinegar (1.5 Tbsp.)
- Coconut cream (2-3 Tbsp.)

- Nutritional yeast (2 Tbsp.)

- Sea salt (1.5 tsp)

Sauce:

- Cassava flour (2 Tbsp.)

- Olive oil (1 Tbsp.)

- Veggie stock (.75 c)

- Coconut cream (2 Tbsp.)

- Sea salt (.5 tsp)

- Parsley (a handful, roughly chopped)

Instructions:

1. Process mushrooms, garlic, and onion in a food processor until finely chopped.

2. Warm oil in a pan then cooks onion mixture until brown. Add in nutritional yeast, vinegar, and cook for 5 minutes.

3. Add in cream and parsley, then turn off the heat.

4. Prepare your dough. Mix all dry ingredients and make a well in the middle. Add in hot water and knead together until well incorporated.

5. Roll dough into a thin sheet. Then put in lumps of filling of dough, with plenty of room around them. Add a second sheet of dough on top and cut and seal with a pizza cutter and a fork.

6. Cook ravioli for 3-5 minutes on boiling water until they float to the surface.

7. Create your cream sauce. Make a roux with flour. Then, add in veggie stock, whisking constantly. Add in salt and cream, then mix well. Plate with ravioli drizzled with sauce and topped with parsley.

__Aloo Gobi__

Serves: 8

Time: 45 minutes

Ingredients:

- Carrot (12 medium, chopped)

- Cauliflower (2 heads, chopped

- Cilantro (2 bunches, chopped)

- Coconut oil (half c.)

- Garlic (6 cloves, minced)

- Ginger (2 Tbsp., grated)

- Ginger powder (4 tsp)

- Onion (2 small, chopped)

- Sea salt (4 tsp)

- Taro root (3 lbs., chopped)

- Turmeric (4 tsp)

- Water (1 c)

Instructions:

1. Begin by preparing your vegetables. Cauliflower needs to be chopped into bite-sized bits. Onions should be in julienned strips. Carrots must be chopped into bites. Taro should be similar to a carrot.

2. Begin warming up your oil in a saucepan. Then, when the coconut oil is melted, toss in all aromatics (onion,

ginger, turmeric, cinnamon). Cook until onions are translucent.

3. Toss in other veggies, as well as the herbs and seasonings left out.

4. Fill in water, then allow it to simmer for 20 minutes. Wait for carrots to become tender.

5. Serve over rice or cauliflower rice. Enjoy!

Chapter 10:
Creating Your Own Meal Plan

So, at this point, you've seen several of the meal plan options that you have for yourself. You see exactly how you can begin to manage your diet. You can choose to enjoy these foods that have been provided to you, or you could also choose to step away from these recipes and start putting together your own plans. As you have read so far, you've got a solid feel for the kinds of foods that you can enjoy and the kinds of foods that are going to be problematic. You can see that there are certain foods that you simply must avoid. Certain foods are more likely to harm you than do anything well, and because of that, you have to be mindful. You have to choose out foods that are loaded up with your anti-inflammatory foods. You want to ensure that you are choosing out foods that will help your body to heal, and the best way to do so is to manage your meal plan.

So far, you know that you are on the right track. You know that you are going to be eating foods that will help you, and you know that you have to create your own meal plan. This chapter is going to help you to understand in more depth how to create your own meal plan that you can actually utilize. And as a bonus, you will be shown two sample meal plans that you can use to help yourself to understand what your diet will look like. You will see that your diet doesn't have to be bad—it just has to work for you. You can make this diet work well for you and for your family as well.

Before we begin to understand what your diet is going to look like and before setting up your meal plan, we will first take the time to consider what kinds of foods and in which kinds of ratios you should be enjoying. This will help you to get a better understanding of the various foods that you are consuming, and by doing so, you should be able to balance out your diet.

Hopefully, this chapter will give you that solid understanding of everything you need to include in your diet. It should help you to understand the foods that you consume and how they can help you as well. So, are you ready? Pull out your pencil and notebook so you can follow along and create your own custom meal plan!

The Anti-Inflammatory Meal Plan Spread

To begin, we will first talk about the foods that you should be consuming and in which ratios. The truth is, when you follow this diet, you will be choosing out foods that are going to benefit you. You are choosing out foods that you know are going to help your body heal, but that requires you to follow a certain balance of the foods that you consume.

When you want to follow the anti-inflammatory diet, you want o keep the foods that you eat balanced out carefully. You want to ensure that you are mindfully choosing out dishes that are going to benefit you, and the sooner that you can do so, the better. We will first address foods that you should be eating in your own personal diet. Then, we will also be taking a look at how your plates should look at any point in time. When you follow along, you should find that you can better control your diet and ensure that it is kept healthy.

The Mediterranean food pyramid

The Mediterranean diet tells you the kinds of foods that you should be consuming on a regular. As you follow along with this diet, you should find that you can address the right kinds of foods. When you go through the process of following the Mediterranean food pyramid, you help yourself to consume primarily anti-inflammatory foods in ratios that are beneficial to you. Consider the following foods:

Daily foods:

- *Bread, grains, potatoes:* These foods will make up the bulk of your calories, but no the bulk of your space. You want to get in between 3 and 6 servings of whole grains and starches whenever possible.

- *Fruits:* Fruits are good for you to enjoy as well. They will provide you a quick, sweet treat that you can enjoy. Generally speaking, you want to eat several different fruits of various colors to ensure that you are getting that diversity that you need. These are going to make up roughly three servings per day.

- *Vegetables:* The biggest part of your diet is going to be veggies. Again, you want to vary the color to ensure that you get the nutritional requirements for your day. You should eat at least three servings of vegetables per day, and they should always take up the most space on your plate.

- *Beans, legumes, and nuts:* These foods are eaten in small amounts daily. You don't need much—after all, they are full of fat. However, if you are following a vegetarian plan, you need the source of both fat and protein that you can get from them. You should get at least once serving per day.

- *Cheese and yogurt:* If you are not following a vegan diet, you will want to introduce small amounts of cheese and yogurt into your diet unless you discover that you are sensitive to these ingredients. They will help you to stay strong and load up on the protein that you need. You should get up to one serving of dairy per day.

- *Olive oil:* Olive oil becomes a staple in this diet. It is one of the most important sources of fat that you will be enjoying. Generally speaking, you should consume between 1 and 4 tablespoons of olive oil per day, depending upon the meals that you are consuming.

Weekly foods

- *Fish:* As long as you are not following the vegan or vegetarian plans, fish should be a major source of protein for you. You want between 1 and 3 servings per week of fish in your diet to get those healthy fats to keep your body thriving.

- *Poultry:* Like fish, poultry (including chicken and turkey) should be consumed between 1 and 3 times per week as well to get that protein spread.

- *Eggs:* Like fish and poultry, you should enjoy whole eggs up to 3 times per week. But, you can also consume egg whites freely without many limitations if they are a part of your diet.

- *Sweets:* If you are enjoying sweets on this diet, you want to consume them no more than once per week. You will still need to be mindful of which sweets you consume and try to keep the added sugar levels low. This will help you to be certain that you are avoiding inflammation.

Rarely consumed foods:

- *Red meat:* If you are consuming meats, you should cut red meat down to as little as possible. These foods are highly inflammatory, and you should have them in extreme moderation.

- *Processed foods:* Like red meat, you want to reduce these as much as possible to keep your body healthy.

The Harvard ratio

When it comes to planning out your food at any point in time, you can usually keep it simple by remembering the Harvard ratio. This ratio will help you to guesstimate the right ratios of food when you are plating your food. This helps immensely with plating food, especially if you are somewhere that is not your home where you have complete control over the foods you are eating. The Harvard ratio tells you that your plate should be balanced as follows:

- ½ plate should be vegetables

- ¼ plate should be whole grains or starch

- ¼ plate should be protein

With those ratios in mind, start thinking about the foods that you will eat. Figure out which foods you will be committing yourself to so that you can be certain that you are always eating foods that work for you. The more that you work on consuming those healthier foods, the better you will do.

Following this ratio will help you greatly as well. This ratio that has been provided to you will help you to figure out which foods are going to be useful. They help you to see the foods that you will be consuming so you can be certain that you are on the right track. When you fill your own personal plate to these ratios, you know that, for the most part, you are picking out food options that are going to be beneficial to you.

You should, for the most part, find that filling your plate in this manner is actually quite balanced. You will be able to turn any meal set to allow you to feed yourself and keep yourself full and healthy.

Sample 2-Week Meal Plan

With everything in mind, you may be interested in understanding seeing what a recipe plan might look like. Remember, you want to make sure that you've got the foods that will keep your meals perfectly balanced. To give yourself a sample meal plan, consider following this meal plan for two weeks to get a look at how you can begin to heal your body.

Week 1

Day 1:

Breakfast: Turmeric scrambled eggs

Lunch: Lemon herb chicken and potatoes

Dinner: Mediterranean mahi mahi

Day 2:

Breakfast: Breakfast casserole

Lunch: Mediterranean salad with grilled chicken

Dinner: Greek stuffed mushrooms

Day 3:

Breakfast: Banana and blueberry pancakes

Lunch: Coconut curry

Dinner: Roasted salmon with Brussels sprouts

Day 4:

Breakfast: Overnight oats

Lunch: Mulligatawny

Dinner: Slow cooked Mediterranean chicken

Day 5:

Breakfast: Overnight oats

Lunch: Harissa pasta

Dinner: Leftover night!

Day 6:

Breakfast: Breakfast casserole

Lunch: Easy Mediterranean pasta salad

Dinner: Mushroom raviolis

Day 7:

Breakfast: Banana and blueberry pancakes

Lunch: Chicken and chickpea soup

Dinner: Turmeric baked salmon

Week 2:

Day 1:

Breakfast: Instant pot quinoa

Lunch: Slow cooked brisket

Dinner: Slow cooked Mediterranean chicken

Day 2:

Breakfast: Instant pot quinoa

Lunch: Slow cooked brisket

Dinner: Mediterranean chicken and couscous wraps

Day 3:

Breakfast: Avocado and kale omelet

Lunch: Slow cooked brisket

Dinner:

Snack:

Day 4:

Breakfast: Breakfast casserole

Lunch: Chow Mein

Dinner: Shrimp stir fry

Day 5:

Breakfast: Tropical breakfast bowl

Lunch: Chow Mein

Dinner: Leftover night!

Day 6:

Breakfast: Apple cinnamon rolls

Lunch: Curried cauliflower rice

Dinner: Loaded baked potato soup

Day 7:

Breakfast: Apple cinnamon rolls

Lunch: Baked cod

Dinner: Chicken and kale curry

Sample Vegetarian Meal Plan

Of course, if you are vegetarian, you might want to change up your meal plan a bit more to ensure that it works well for the foods that you are going to be eating as well. You will need to ensure that the diet plan that you come up with is going to provide you with plenty of nourishment without being too bland or repetitive. This will help you to ensure that the diet that you enjoy is perfect.

Week 1

Day 1:

Breakfast: Avocado and kale omelet

Lunch: Chow Mein

Dinner: Greek stuffed mushrooms

Day 2:

Breakfast: Instant Pot cinnamon porridge

Lunch: Curried cauliflower rice

Dinner: Vegetarian zucchini lasagna rolls

Day 3:

Breakfast: Cauliflower oatmeal

Lunch: Ratatouille

Dinner: Cheesy artichoke and spinach stuffed squash

Day 4:

Breakfast: Tigernut granola

Lunch: Mulligatawny

Dinner: Bean and spinach soup

Day 5:

Breakfast: Banana coconut bread

Lunch: Spinach tacos

Dinner: Leftover night!

Day 6:

Breakfast: Lemon waffles

Lunch: Harissa pasta

Dinner: Vegan Mediterranean pasta

Day 7:

Breakfast: Banana and blueberry pancakes

Lunch: Chow Mein

Dinner: Miso tofu stir fry

Week 2:

Day 1:

Breakfast: Overnight oats

Lunch: Mediterranean pasta salad

Dinner: Sweet potato cauliflower soup

Day 2:

Breakfast: Overnight oats

Lunch: Harissa pasta

Dinner: Mushroom raviolis

Day 3:

Breakfast: Sweet potato cookies

Lunch: Moroccan lentil soup

Dinner: Greek stuffed mushrooms

Day 4:

Breakfast: Pumpkin bagels

Lunch: Coconut curry

Dinner: Vegetarian zucchini lasagna rolls

Day 5:

Breakfast: Banana coconut bread

Lunch: Curried cauliflower rice

Dinner: Leftover night!

Day 6:

Breakfast: Banana coconut bread

Lunch: Coconut curry

Dinner: Aloo gobi

Day 7:

Breakfast: Veggie breakfast muffins

Lunch: Mulligatawny

Dinner: Vegan Mediterranean pasta

Chapter 11:
Bonus Tips and Tricks to Sticking to Your Diet

Sticking to diets can be quite difficult if you don't know what to do. It can be hard to have the right mindset, the right structure, the right habits, and the right support to ensure that you do stick to what you need at all times. However, if you know what you are doing, you should be able to get through with ease. Ultimately, being able to stick to your diet will help you immensely. Especially with this particular diet and knowing that you are eating to keep your body healthy, you need to have the ability to keep yourself on track. If you want to stick to your diet and if you want to ensure that your body begins to heal, you want to figure out how to stick to your diet. All you have to do to make that happen is to ensure that you keep these tips in mind.

Remember that when you are following this diet, you will need to find a way to ensure that you are on the right track. You need to ensure that you are giving yourself that positivity, and when you do this the right way, you can get yourself to stick to the success that you are looking for. All you will have to do is ensure that you are actively working toward bettering yourself. These tricks and tips will help you greatly. You can do it! Yes, you might have some dietary limitations, but you can still have a delicious diet and enjoy your food as well. All you have to do is make sure that you build the right mindset.

Be Realistic

The most important rule to any dietary change that you make is to remember to be realistic about whatever changes you do make. Ultimately, remembering what you are doing and being realistic about how long it will take for this diet to work will help you not only to curb any disappointment that you might feel if you decide that this diet is not actually working but also keep you on track. After all, if you acknowledge that it takes time for your body to heal from eating inflammatory food, you are going to naturally be less inclined to actually eat those inflammatory food options. You will be more motivated to keep yourself and your diet on track just so you do not have to wait so long to ever actually heal from them.

Having that realistic attitude helps you to remember that ultimately, just because things are tough at the moment, or just because you feel like things aren't proceeding fast enough doesn't mean you should quit. You are committing to a healthier lifestyle. You are committing to being healthier in general, and that means that you will need to be able to treat yourself well. You will need to be able to remind yourself that your dietary choices are there for a reason and that you don't want to forget about why.

Follow Your Motivations

That brings us to our second tip for maintaining your diet—reminding yourself of your motivations so you can acknowledge exactly why you are trying to keep yourself on track. Are you on this diet because you want to be healthier? Are you trying to figure out which foods you can and cannot eat? Are you on this diet to try to heal your body and get relief from whatever has been hurting you? There are all sorts of reasons that people choose to follow those anti-inflammatory diets, and when you acknowledge why you choose to follow it, you will find yourself doing so much better. You will be able to help yourself to feel better and more on track with your own diet if you can remember to follow your motivations. At the end of the day, you want to be able to keep yourself on track.

Consider keeping a sort of memento handy for yourself to provide yourself with that added benefit of maintaining your intention. When you start feeling tempted to grab that food that isn't going to be any good for you, you can then tell yourself not to. Your memento that you use, such as a picture of your child playing soccer if you are trying to take this diet into consideration specifically because of the fact that you suffer from arthritis and you want to be able to play with them after you can reduce down some of the swelling and pain. Maybe you want to be able to go out without having to constantly worry about where the bathroom is. There are all sorts of reasons that you probably have to pursue your own diet and the sooner that you can address those reasons and remind yourself to follow them, the better.

Keep Healthy Foods in Stock

Of course, one of the best ways that you can keep yourself on track with your diet is to simply always maintain healthy foods in stock. If you want to be able to eat the foods that you know are going to benefit you, you will need to ensure that you have those foods in stock. When you do your shopping, you should keep in mind that by keeping the healthiest options for you in stock, you actually reduce the chances of you consuming something unhealthy.

If you do buy foods that are unhealthy or are inflammatory, you run the risk of consuming them just due to the fact that you have them. If you have other family members that enjoy those foods, consider making it a point to only keep those foods in stock for those people, and then keep them separate from the food that you are consuming. When you do this, you will give yourself that degree of separation to keep yourself on track. Out of sight, out of mind, after all.

Avoid All or Nothing Thoughts

Remember as well that you need to avoid all or nothing thoughts. If you found that you accidentally consumed something that you shouldn't have, instead of getting upset about it or deciding just to binge because clearly your diet was ruined anyway, simply get right back to working on yourself. You want to ensure that you are actively choosing to stick to your healthy diet as much as possible. Did you cave and eat a cupcake at your work party? That's okay—just move on. Just keep pushing yourself forward and remember that ultimately, you need to stay healthy and get yourself back on track. Instead of considering the day of eating ruined anyway, just let it go and get back on track. Start making healthy choices again. While your body will probably not appreciate the introduction of anything inflammatory, you can get yourself back on track sooner rather than later and feel better than you expected to. This will help you immensely and is an essential way for you to get moving healthily.

Pay Attention When Eating Out

One thing that you need to remember is that when you are eating out, it is hard to have full transparency on what you are consuming. When you eat out, there can be all sorts of hidden ingredients in the dishes, and that can be a big problem. When you are on this diet, you need to remember the dishes may not actually be anti-inflammatory friendly. This is why it was so crucial to have that list of inflammatory foods as well as the list of anti-inflammatory options so you could focus on the foods that you know are going to be good for you. You want to ensure that the foods that you enjoy are actually anti-inflammatory. When you know that list of foods that are safer for you, you will be able to consume them. You will also be able to ask about dishes on the menu that you are curious about. By learning about the dishes in them, you will then be able to keep yourself healthier. You will be able to turn out the dishes that have the inflammatory ingredients included, meaning that you have the perfect option to keep up with yourself and the food choices you make.

Accountability

A great way to help yourself make those lifestyle changes is to find someone else to help you. You want to figure out if you can find people to stick to your diet with you. You might want to find out if there are groups of people around you that will help you stick to your diet. You could, for example, bring other people into your diet. Or, you could make it a point to find a support group. If you have an autoimmune disorder, you could potentially find groups of people also suffering from that disorder as well. These support groups could be full of people that are keeping this diet in mind as well.

Sometimes, dieting is difficult when you don't have other people working with you. Because of that, it can be a great thing for you to actively find ways to work with others. When you get to work with other people, you have other people who understand when you mention that you miss some food that you had been eating before. You have people who will support you, and they will also help you to keep yourself accountable.

Change Your Mindset

Another key way that you can consider is changing your mindset. Make sure that you've got the right mindset to approach your dietary changes as well. This means that you must be determined and dedicated. Dieting takes time and effort, even if you are not actively trying to lose weight. However, keep in mind that when it comes time to diet, you must ensure that you are doing so in an effective manner. You want to make sure that, when you do the diet, you are doing so with the right mindset so you can keep yourself on track even when the going gets tough. You want to ensure that when you are listening to the people around you, you are actively working to better yourself. You need to want to be on a diet, or it won't work.

When you are going into dieting, remember that you should have it framed positively. You don't *have* to eat healthily; you *get to* eat healthily. See that simple change in mindset? That little shift in mindset can actually help you to feel better. It will remind you that you can and will be able to stick to your diet because you chose to do it. You are reminding yourself that your diet is a good thing ad that you are lucky to be able to stick to it in the first place. Reminding yourself that you are in a position of being lucky rather than in a position of simply having to do something will make it easier. This is because you are framing your diet as something that you want. You are framing it as something positive. You are making yourself know that what you wanted more than anything was the success in this diet, and that will help you. It will become automatic over time.

Teach Yourself That Hunger Is Not an Emergency

Another key point to remember is that hunger is not actually the emergency that you might feel like it is. Most people can skip a meal without much of a problem. While there are a few exceptions to this, and while some people may find that dieting and skipping meals can actually be highly detrimental when not managed carefully, such as people with Type 1 Diabetes, most of us can get by without lunch every now and then. At most, it is simply unpleasant and uncomfortable. However, it is nothing more than that—it is an inconvenience, and that is it. When you diet for yourself, you might lose steam just because you feel like it is uncomfortable. However, remember that your diet is not all bad. Remember that even if you feel hungry, sometimes when you follow your diet, you are just hungry. Hunger every now and then is not anything to worry about.

To help you reiterate this point, consider skipping lunch a couple of days. Get through the hunger. Show yourself that even if you are hungry sometimes, you don't have anything to worry about. This will help you to remember that if you do go out one day and realize that you are absolutely ravenous, you don't have to actually head out and eat anything immediately. You can wait until you get home to avoid ordering takeout or buying snacks that may be problematic for you.

Recognize the Difference Between Hunger and Cravings

Consider as well that sometimes, when you think you are hungry, you are really just craving something. Usually, when that temptation to eat something hits, it is more along the lines of emotional eating than actually needing to consume anything in the first place. Maybe you chose to eat something to alleviate your stress or because you were angry or anxious. When you are in a poor state of mind, you might tell yourself that you really do need that extra scoop of ice cream or that greasy cheeseburger. It has less to do with you actually being hungry and more to do with you simply wanting to indulge. You run into this issue where you struggle to actually stick to your diet simply because your emotions rule you.

So, what is the difference between hunger and cravings? Simple. When you are truly hungry, you will feel it in your stomach. You will find yourself feeling tired, weak, or even suffering from a headache, and usually, you will not have eaten in a while before that hunger strikes. You can usually satisfy that hunger simply with any sort of healthy food.

Cravings, on the other hand, are usually specifically for foods that you know will make you feel better. They may be for sweets or fatty foods, both of which trigger those feel-good endorphins in the brain. They also tend to get stronger when you feel negative. They are felt more in the mouth and throat than in the stomach—it is that drive to get something to satisfy your mouth rather than your stomach.

The good news is that cravings can be beaten. Hunger has to be satisfied, but craving can be ignored, or you can also simply distract yourself from it. When you know that you have a craving, the best thing that you can do is simply distract yourself from them and do something more productive that is going to help you to do better and stick to your diet. You could, for example, try to make yourself feel better, or you could work out or do something unrelated. Try drinking a glass of water as well if you want to be able to distance yourself from your craving while still satisfying that need for something in your mouth.

Set the Habits

Finally, when you want to stick to your diet, you want to set the right habits ahead of time. By setting those good habits in stone, you can make it easier to follow your diet. We are creatures of habit, after all, and the sooner that you realize this and start working with it, the better. The more that you make something habitual, the more likely you are to actually stick to it. The more that you make those healthy choices, the easier it will get for you to make them as well. This is essential—if you want to be able to eat those healthier foods for yourself, the best thing that you can do is make it habitual. After all, so much of our taste preferences simply come from habit. While sugar may taste good, for those who do not habitually eat it, it can actually feel overwhelmingly sweet, and they actually prefer to avoid it rather than consuming it. When you consider this point and stick to it, you can actually begin to get past your desire for junky foods. You will be able to make your new desire something healthy instead.

Conclusion

If you have been living with inflammation, chances are you have been struggling for far longer than you probably want to admit. You probably don't want to continue suffering, but if you don't know what you are doing, you are going to struggle to eliminate the problem. You want to make sure that you know how you can heal yourself. You want to know what you can do to eliminate that inflammation for yourself, and ultimately, through reading this book, you will be able to figure it all out. Hopefully, after reading everything that you have read, you have a better understanding of everything that you will need.

When you work on yourself, and you work to heal yourself, you should be able to figure out how to eliminate the inflammation in your life. Being able to keep the inflammation levels down is imperative if you want to heal. We have spent this entire book so far working on teaching you how you can heal yourself. The more that you do it, the better you will do. The more that you work on providing yourself the right situation to heal yourself, the better you will do.

When you work hard, you will be able to heal your body, little by little. When you implement the various information in this book and begin to create your own meal plans, you can start recovering with ease. You just have to know what you are doing and work hard to put it to good work. The more that you do so, the better. So, start creating your meal plans. What are you waiting for? It's time to head up and begin figuring out which of the recipes provided to you are the ones that you want to enjoy. It is time to start experimenting with all of the various recipes that you've got given to you. The more that you try these various recipes, the better you will feel.

So, from here, the next thing that you will need to do is figure out how you can start implementing your foods. Remember to start cutting out those inflammatory foods. Remember to start working to provide yourself with the best ways to heal yourself. It is time to start remembering to work on your meal plan and planning out your shopping lists.

If you start to feel discouraged, remember that this diet is all about healing yourself. It is there for a reason, and you should make it a point to remember this. You should be applying yourself seriously and working to give yourself that success that you are looking for. Remind yourself of what you are working for. Remind yourself of why this diet is so essential to yourself, and keep strong. Remember to maintain your own support. Remember to be patient with yourself and patient with the results as well. Before you know it, you should be able to discover that, though restrictive, this diet will help you immensely. It is healthy, and it is healing as well. You can alleviate the inflammation that you have had in your life and begin to heal once and for all.

If you need some more information or more inspiration for meals, consider taking a look at some of the most common anti-inflammatory diets that are out there for more recipes. You could, for example, take a look at the various meals in the Mediterranean diet. You could look at the Sirtfood diet, which features many anti-inflammatory foods thanks to its emphasis on so many antioxidant-rich foods within it. You could turn to all sorts of other foods that you know are going to give yourself that healing boost as well. You could take a look at the autoimmune protocol diet as well, which closely follows paleo recipes. All you have to do is know where to look, and you can find yourself being exposed to so many other recipes that you know will be beneficial to you. You just have to try!

And finally, if you found that the recipes provided to you within this book have been enjoyable, healthy, and easy to make, consider heading over to Amazon to leave a review. Those reviews may be enough to sway someone else like you to read through this book and begin healing their own body as well. This will help you greatly. And, your opinions and feedback about the recipes can help immensely as well with ensuring that future content is also quality content! Good luck out there, and Bon appetite!